OXFORD MEDICAL PUBLICATIONS

Urogynaecology

T0177612

Oxford Specialist Handbooks in Obstetrics and Gynaecology
Series editor | Sally Collins

Obstetric Medicine
Charlotte Frise and Sally Collins

Urogynaecology
Helen Jefferis and Natalia Price

Oxford Specialist Handbooks in Obstetrics and Gynaecology
Urogynaecology

Helen Jefferis

Consultant Urogynaecologist
John Radcliffe Hospital,
Oxford University Hospitals NHS Foundation Trust
Oxford, UK

Natalia Price

Consultant Urogynaecologist
John Radcliffe Hospital,
Oxford University Hospitals NHS Foundation Trust
Oxford, UK

OXFORD
UNIVERSITY PRESS

OXFORD
UNIVERSITY PRESS

Great Clarendon Street, Oxford, OX2 6DP,
United Kingdom

Oxford University Press is a department of the University of Oxford.
It furthers the University's objective of excellence in research, scholarship,
and education by publishing worldwide. Oxford is a registered trade mark of
Oxford University Press in the UK and in certain other countries

Published in the United States of America by Oxford University Press
198 Madison Avenue, New York, NY 10016, United States of America

British Library Cataloguing in Publication Data
Data available

Library of Congress Catalogin in Publication Data
Data available

ISBN 978–0–19–882906–5

Printed in Great Britain by
Ashford Colour Press Ltd, Gosport, Hampshire

Preface

Welcome to the first edition of this Oxford Handbook, which uses the familiar Oxford Handbook format to enable the reader to easily navigate around evidence-based urogynaecology topics. Wherever possible web links to the latest national guidance are included for reference and additional reading.

Whilst the content will be particularly relevant for gynaecology doctors undertaking subspecialty or ATSM level urogynaecology training, we also anticipate it being useful for anyone with an interest in pelvic floor dysfunction, including urologists, colorectal specialists and physiotherapists. This book also describes pelvic floor conditions that may be encountered by any generalist in the field and covers the knowledge required for the MRCOG.

We hope this will be a valuable pocket-sized aid to assessment and management of simple and complex pelvic floor disorders.

Contents

Symbols and abbreviations *ix*

1	Anatomy and physiology	1
2	Assessment of the urinary tract	7
3	Lower urinary tract conditions	27
4	Pelvic organ prolapse	57
5	Urology	83
6	Colorectal	111
7	Neurology	127
8	Pregnancy and childbirth	137
9	Age and the pelvic floor	147
10	Laparoscopic urogynaecology	155
11	Miscellaneous	165

Index *175*

Symbols and abbreviations

❶	Warning
▶	Important
♒	Online reference
↑	Increased
↓	Decreased
⮌	Cross reference
ASC	ambulatory surgery centre
ATSM	Advanced Training Skills Modules [RCOG]
BCG	Bacillus Calmette-Guérin
BMI	body mass index
BPS	bladder pain syndrome
BSUG	British Society of Urogynaecology
CIC	clean intermittent catheterization
CNS	central nervous system
CS	caesarean section
CT	computed tomography
DMSO	dimethyl sulfoxide
DO	detrusor overactivity
DVT	deep venous thrombosis
EAS	external anal sphincter
EMG	electromyogram
EUA	examination under anaesthesia
FDA	US Food and Drug Administration
GA	general anaesthetic
GI	gastrointestinal
HRT	hormone replacement therapy
IAS	internal anal sphincter
ICIQ-VS	International Consultation on Incontinence Questionnaire–Vaginal Symptoms
ICS	International Continence Society
IV	intravenous
IVU	intravenous urogram
LSC	laparoscopic sacrocolpopexy
LUTS	lower urinary tract symptoms
MDT	multidisciplinary team
MHRA	Medicines and Healthcare products Regulatory Agency
MRI	magnetic resonance imaging
MS	multiple sclerosis
MSU	midstream specimen of urine
NICE	National Institute for Health and Care Excellence
OASI	obstetric anal sphincter injury
ODS	obstructed defaecation syndrome
OP	occiput posterior
PCOS	polycystic ovary syndrome
PID	pelvic inflammatory disease
POP	pelvic organ prolapse
POP-Q	Pelvic Organ Prolapse Quantification
PTNS	percutaneous tibial nerve stimulation
PV	per vaginam
RCOG	Royal College of Obstetricians and Gynaecologists
RCT	randomized controlled trial
RVF	rectovaginal fistula
SLE	systemic lupus erythematosus
SNRI	serotonin and norepinephrine reuptake inhibitor
SNS	sacral nerve stimulation
SPC	suprapubic catheter
SSF	sacrospinous ligament fixation
STAMP	sutured transanal mucosectomy and plication
STARR	stapled transanal resection of rectum
STI	sexually transmitted infection
SUI	stress urinary incontinence
TB	tuberculosis
TVT	tension-free vaginal tape
TWOC	trial without catheter
UPP	urethral pressure profilometry
USS	ultrasound scan
UTI	urinary tract infection
VVF	vesicovaginal fistula

Anatomy and physiology

Anatomy of the urinary tract 2
Anatomy of the pelvic floor 4
Control of micturition 6

Anatomy of the urinary tract

Ureter
- 25–30cm in length
- Transport urine by peristalsis
- Retroperitoneal.

Course
- Runs on the anteromedial aspect of the psoas muscle
- Crossed by the ovarian vessels
- Crosses over the bifurcation of the common iliac artery
- At the true pelvis, turns forwards and medial, passing lateral to the uterosacral ligaments and running through the base of the broad ligament
- Crossed by the uterine artery ('water under the bridge')
- Runs 1.5cm lateral to the cervix
- Enters the bladder at the trigone at an oblique angle to prevent reflux.

Bladder
- Retroperitoneal
- A muscular reservoir
- Formed of three layers of muscle known collectively as the detrusor
- Extends upwards and outwards as it fills
- Lined by transitional epithelium (urothelium): high resistance barrier function, highly hormonally sensitive.

Trigone
- Triangular region of the bladder defined by the urethral opening and the ureteric orifices.

Urethra
- 4cm long
- Richly vascular spongy cylinder immediately related to anterior vaginal wall
- Lined by transitional epithelium proximally, squamous epithelium distally
- Internal urethral sphincter—smooth muscle fibres, kept under tonic contraction by sympathetic fibres of hypogastric nerve
- Striated 'external sphincter' (compressor urethrae)—distal two-thirds of urethra, innervated by somatic fibres of pudendal nerve and under voluntary control
- Vascularity helps maintain urethral closure.

▶ Vascularity and hence closure is adversely affected by hypo-oestrogenic states.

Anatomy of the pelvic floor

▶ The 'pelvic floor' is a term given to the muscular and fascial structures providing support to the pelvic viscera, vagina, rectum, and urethra.
See Fig. 1.1.

Pelvic floor muscles

Refers to levator ani and coccygeus, which form a funnel shaped sheet of muscle.

- Levator ani is made up of three components:
  - Puborectalis—forms a U-shaped sling around the rectum and is most important at maintaining faecal continence. Relaxes to allow defaecation
  - Pubococcygeus—the main constituent of levator ani
  - Iliococcygeus—contraction elevates the pelvic floor and anorectal canal
- Innervated by the pudendal nerve (roots S2–4).

Role of the pelvic floor muscles
- Support abdominal and pelvic viscera
- Resist increased intra-abdominal pressure
- Urinary and faecal continence.

Levels of vaginal support

The uterus and vagina are suspended from the pelvic side walls by endopelvic fascial attachments, providing support at three levels:

- *Level 1*: The cervix and upper third of the vagina are supported by the cardinal and uterosacral ligaments, suspending the cervix and top of the vagina from the pelvic side wall and sacrum.
- *Level 2*: The middle of the vagina is attached laterally to the pelvic side walls (arcus tendineus) by endopelvic fascial condensation.
- *Level 3*: The lower third of the vagina is supported by the levator ani muscles and the perineal body.

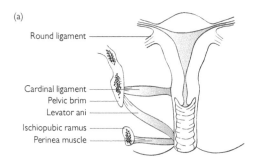

(a)

Round ligament

Cardinal ligament
Pelvic brim
Levator ani
Ischiopubic ramus
Perinea muscle

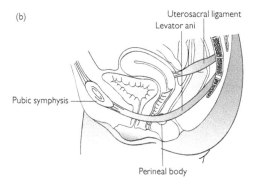

(b)

Uterosacral ligament
Levator ani

Pubic symphysis

Perineal body

Fig. 1.1 (a) Coronal view of the pelvis, showing cardinal ligaments and levator ani.
(b) Lateral view of the pelvis, showing the uterosacral ligaments and levator ani.

Reprinted from Impey L and Child T (2012) *Obstetrics and Gynaecology* Oxford: Wiley-Blackwell
publishing, with permission from John Wiley & Sons

Control of micturition

Requires coordinated contraction and relaxation of the bladder and urethral sphincter, under the control of complex pathways in the brain, spinal cord, and peripheral nervous system.

Storage phase

Throughout bladder filling, the parasympathetic innervation of the detrusor is inhibited and the urethral sphincter is contracted, preventing urinary leakage.

Continence centres in cerebral cortex
↓
Pontine continence centre
↓
Sympathetic nuclei in spinal cord
↓
Sympathetic hypogastric nerve (L1–2)
↓↓
Relaxes detrusor muscle   Contracts urethra

Compliance

As the bladder fills, intravesical pressure does not rise, meaning that urethral pressure is greater than the intravesical pressure and so continence is maintained.

Voiding phase

Afferent signals from stretching of the bladder wall ascend through the spinal cord to the pontine micturition centre then cerebral cortex.

Voluntary decision to urinate
↓
Neurons of the pontine micturition centre fire and excite sacral preganglionic neurons
↓   ↓
Pelvic nerve (S2–4)   Inhibit Onuf's nucleus
↓   ↓
Acetylcholine release   Reduced sympathetic stimulation
↓   ↓
Detrusor contraction   Internal urethral sphincter relaxation

---

▶ In addition, there is a conscious reduction in external urethral sphincter contraction.

Assessment of the urinary tract

Symptoms and definitions 8
Initial assessment of the patient 10
Baseline investigations 12
Imaging of the urinary tract 12
Cystoscopy 14
Urodynamic tests 16
Uroflowmetry 18
Cystometry 20
Additional urodynamic tests 24
Urethral pressure profilometry 26

Symptoms and definitions

The following are ICS agreed terminology.

Storage symptoms

- *Daytime frequency*—complaint that micturition occurs more frequently than previously deemed normal by the woman.
- *Nocturia*—complaint of interruption of sleep one or more times because of the need to micturate. Each void is preceded and followed by sleep.
- *Urgency*—complaint of a sudden, compelling desire to void which is difficult to defer.
- *Urinary incontinence*—complaint of involuntary loss of urine.
- *Stress urinary incontinence (SUI)*—complaint of involuntary loss of urine on effort or physical exertion including sporting activities, etc., or on sneezing or coughing.
- *Urgency urinary incontinence*—complaint of involuntary loss of urine associated with urgency.
- *Mixed urinary incontinence*—complaint of involuntary loss of urine associated with urgency and also with effort or physical exertion, or on sneezing or coughing.
- *Overactive bladder (OAB) syndrome*—urinary urgency, usually accompanied by frequency and nocturia, with or without urgency urinary incontinence, in the absence of urinary tract infection or other obvious pathology.
- *Nocturnal enuresis*—complaint of involuntary urinary loss of urine which occurs during sleep.
- *Unconscious (insensible) urinary incontinence*—complaint of involuntary loss of urine unaccompanied by either urgency or stress incontinence provocative factors. The only awareness of the incontinence episode is the feeling of wetness due to the urine.
- *Coital incontinence*—complaint of involuntary loss of urine with coitus. This symptom might be further divided into that occurring with penetration and that occurring at orgasm.

Voiding symptoms

- *Poor stream*—complaint of a urinary stream perceived as slower or more interrupted compared to that previously experienced or in comparison to others.
- *Intermittent stream*—is the term used when the individual describes urine flow which stops and starts, on one or more occasions, during micturition.
- *Hesitancy*—complaint of a delay in initiating micturition.
- *Straining to void*—complaint of the need to make an intensive effort (by abdominal straining, Valsalva, or suprapubic pressure) to either initiate, maintain, or improve the urinary stream.
- *Need to immediately re-void*—complaint that further micturition is necessary soon after passing urine.
- *Dysuria*—complaint of burning or other discomfort during micturition. Discomfort may be intrinsic to the lower urinary tract or external (vulvar dysuria).
- *Stranguria*—complaint of micturition which is both painful and difficult.

Postmicturition symptoms
- *Feeling of incomplete (bladder) emptying*—complaint that the bladder does not feel empty after micturition.
- *Postmicturition leakage*—complaint of a further involuntary passage of urine following the completion of micturition.

Lower urinary tract conditions
Urodynamic stress incontinence
- Involuntary leakage during filling cystometry, associated with ↑ intra-abdominal pressure, in the absence of a detrusor muscle contraction.

Detrusor overactivity
- Involuntary detrusor muscle contractions occur during filling cystometry.

Voiding dysfunction
- Abnormally slow and/or incomplete micturition.

Resources
🖰 https://www.ics.org/glossary

Initial assessment of the patient

History of presenting complaint
- Often multiple symptoms
- Key is to establish what is 'most bothersome symptom'
- Identify any red flag symptoms (e.g. haematuria)
- Ask about other symptoms of pelvic floor dysfunction (vaginal, anal, sexual symptoms).

❶ Patients may not volunteer sensitive information unless directly questioned
- Need to identify the impact of symptoms on daily life, work, relationships, etc.

Identify causative factors
- Obstetric history—number and mode of births
- Significant neurological history, e.g. multiple sclerosis
- Relevant medical history, e.g. diabetes
- Previous pelvic surgery
- Review medications
- Review mobility/access to toilet facilities
- Assess fluid intake (type and schedule)
- Ask about bowel habit (constipation compounds urinary problems).

Quality of life
- This is the most important factor to elicit.
- Various validated questionnaires to aid assessment, e.g. King's Health, ICIQ-FLUTS.

Examination
- BMI
- Mobility
- Abdominal palpation—any pelvic mass or distended bladder?
- Inspection of external genitalia—atrophy, chemical irritation from urine
- Assess for prolapse
- Assess pelvic floor strength (Oxford scale)
- Cough test
- Neurological examination if appropriate.

Investigations
Will depend on symptoms—follow investigations in this chapter.

Baseline investigations

- Urinalysis and culture—infection must be excluded before alternative diagnosis is pursued
- Urine cytology—if haematuria present.

(➲ see Chapter 5, Urology, p. 83.)

Postvoid residual

Volume of urine left in the bladder at the completion of micturition.
  May be assessed by:
- Bladder scan
- In-out urethral catheter.

Frequency/volume chart

- Ideally kept for minimum 3 days
- Frequency, timing, and volume of all voids recorded
- All leakage episodes recorded
- Fluid intake (type and time) recorded
- Used to assess functional bladder capacity, voiding behaviour, drinking patterns.

Imaging of the urinary tract
➲ Also see Chapter 5, Urology, p. 90.

Ultrasound
- Assess bladder emptying (postvoid residual)
- Look for congenital anomaly, e.g. duplex kidney
- Detect renal cortical scarring
- Look for pelvic mass.

CT
- Assess for renal masses
- Assess for renal stones
- As part of work up for haematuria.

Cystoscopy

Indications
- Haematuria
- Recurrent UTI
- Bladder pain
- Intraoperative suspicion of urinary tract injury
- Suspicion of fistula
- Suspicion of mesh complication
- In context of certain procedures, e.g. insertion of SPC, colposuspension, retropubic tape.

Equipment
Rigid scope
- 0°, 30°, 70°. 70° needed during retropubic tape insertion to fully visualize bladder neck
- Requires general anaesthesia
- May be more appropriate in context of bladder pain.

Flexible scope
- Performed under local anaesthesia (urethral gel) in outpatient/ diagnostic setting.

Technique for cystoscopy
- Aseptic technique
- Local anaesthetic/antiseptic gel per urethra
- Water used as distension media
- Systematic approach to inspect
  - Bladder mucosa
  - Trigone
  - Number/site of ureteric orifices
  - Urethra
- Make note of volume of water infused (assessment of capacity)
- If assessing for pain, hydrodistension, and second look recommended, which requires GA
- Biopsies may be taken if clinically indicated
- If under GA, drain bladder at end of procedure.

Relevant findings at cystoscopy

Normal findings

- Normal bladder mucosa appears pale pink and smooth.
- The ureteric orifices are found on the posterior wall just past the bladder neck.
- The trigone is a triangular area defined superiorly by the ureteric orifices and inferiorly by the urethral entrance.
- The urethral mucosa is rugose.

Atrophic changes

- Urothelium contains oestrogen receptors and so will change in its absence. The mucosa looks paler with loss of urethral rugae.

Squamous metaplasia

- Trigone looks 'bubbly'.
- Common finding at the trigone with no clinical significance.

Cystitis cystica

- Small subepithelial vesicles.
- Occurs as an inflammatory reaction of urothelium to infection or mechanical irritation.
- Commonly associated with recurrent UTI.

Bladder diverticulum

- May be congenital or acquired.
- Usually incidental finding but may be associated with outlet obstruction and stone formation.

Trabeculation

- Criss-cross appearance due to thickening of the detrusor muscle.
- Seen in bladder outlet obstruction (e.g. procidentia), neurogenic bladder, long-term catheter use.

ⓘ *Carcinoma in situ*

- Has a flat, velvety appearance.
- May be seen in isolation or in association with higher grade disease.

ⓘ *Transitional cell carcinoma*

- Usually appears as a papillary projection.

Urodynamic tests

- This term describes a combination of tests that are used to assess bladder function (i.e. its ability to store and expel urine).
- It is more useful and accurate at diagnosis than symptoms alone which may be misleading.

▶ Urodynamic tests include uroflowmetry, postvoid residual measurement, and cystometry.

Indications

- Mixed or complex symptoms
- Prior to surgical intervention for SUI (although NICE guidance suggests in uncomplicated SUI treatment may be undertaken based on symptoms alone, the authors' preference is to establish a clear diagnosis, exclude provoked DO, and ensure voiding is normal prior to invasive treatment)
- OAB unresponsive to initial conservative and medical treatment
- OAB in the context of neurological disease
- Suspected voiding dysfunction.

Aim of urodynamic tests

- To reproduce symptoms
- To provide a pathophysiological explanation for symptoms
- To answer a specific clinical question (e.g. is there voiding dysfunction?)
- To establish a clear diagnosis
- To determine severity of problem
- To guide therapy.

Uroflowmetry

- The patient attends with a comfortably full bladder and is asked to void in privacy on a commode that incorporates a urinary flow metre.
- This measures voided volume as a function of time and plots it graphically (Fig. 2.1).
- ❶ Interpreting flow rates of <200ml is inaccurate.

Postvoid residual

- Following uroflowmetry a postvoid residual is assessed by bladder scan or by in-out catheter.
- ❶ Volumes of >100ml are considered abnormal.

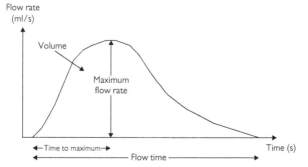

Flow rate (ml/s)

Volume

Maximum flow rate

◄━Time to maximum━► Flow time

Time (s)

Fig. 2.1 Diagrammatic representation of normal urinary flow rate. Voided volume: total volume expelled via the urethra, the area beneath the flow-time curve. Maximum flow rate: maximum measured value of the flow rate. Average flow rate: volume voided divided by the flow time. Flow time: the time over which measurable flow actually occurs.

Reprinted from Collins S et al (2013) Oxford Handbook of Obstetrics and Gynaecology 3rd Edition, Oxford: Oxford University Press, with permission from Oxford University Press

Cystometry

- This is an assessment of bladder function by recording bladder pressures while filling and voiding.
- This requires insertion of a pressure transducer into the bladder (measures intravesical pressure or P_{ves}) and into the rectum (measures intraabdominal pressure or P_{abd}).
- An estimated detrusor pressure (P_{det}) is calculated by subtracting P_{abd} from P_{ves}.
- A filling line is also inserted into the bladder and saline is infused using a peristaltic pump (Fig. 2.2).

▶ The ICS has done much to standardize methodology and interpretation.

❶ Patients should be advised to stop medications affecting bladder function a week prior to the test.

Filling cystometry

Technique

- Saline is infused at a rate of 50ml/min (compared to an average physiological filling rate of 1ml/min).

❶ Faster filling will produce significant artefact.

❶ Slower filling may be required with severe or neurogenic DO.

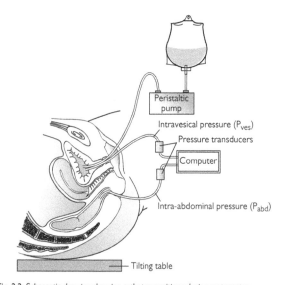

Fig. 2.2 Schematic drawing showing catheter positions during cystometry.

Reprinted from Collins S et al (2013) *Oxford Handbook of Obstetrics and Gynaecology* 3rd Edition, Oxford: Oxford University Press, with permission from Oxford University Press

- Natural filling should have a negligible contribution to bladder volume over the space of a short cystometrogram.
- The patient is asked to cough at regular intervals to check subtraction of the lines.

The patient is asked to tell the examiner when she experiences the following:

- First sensation—when the patient first becomes aware of bladder filling. Typically, at half bladder capacity (150–200ml).
- First desire to void—the first feeling that the woman may wish to void.
- Normal desire to void—the feeling that leads the woman to pass urine at the next convenient moment, but voiding can be delayed if necessary.
- Strong desire to void—the persistent desire to void without the fear of leakage.
- Urgency—sudden compelling desire to void which is difficult to defer.
- Maximum cystometric capacity—the volume when she can no longer delay micturition.

During filling the urodynamicist will observe any pressure changes in P_{det} (see Box 2.1) and relate these to the patient-reported sensation.

Box 2.1 Definition of compliance and contractility

Compliance

This describes the relationship between the change in bladder volume and the change in detrusor pressure. It is measured between two fixed points, usually the start of filling and when cystometric capacity is reached.

$$\text{Compliance} = \frac{\text{Change in volume}}{\text{Change in } P_{det}}$$

During normal bladder filling little or no change is seen (maximum of 30–40ml/cmH$_2$O), which is termed normal compliance.

▶ Poor compliance denotes a gradual rise in detrusor pressure over filling.

Contractility

In patients with a normal bladder, detrusor contractions are inhibited until they are in an acceptable time and place to void.

Results

- Normal detrusor function during filling (previously termed 'stable detrusor'—little or no change in detrusor pressure with filling. There are no involuntary phasic contractions despite provocation.
- DO is the occurrence of involuntary detrusor contractions during filling cystometry. These may:
  - Be spontaneous (usually phasic or wave like)
  - Be provoked (change in position, handwashing, taps on, cough)
  - May or may not be associated with leakage.

Tests of provocation

Once cystometric capacity has been reached the filling line is removed, leaving the pressure transducers in place. Tests of provocation with a full bladder are then used to look for urodynamic stress incontinence. The patient may be asked to cough vigorously, jump, heel rock, etc. Leakage in the absence of a detrusor contraction confirms urodynamic stress incontinence.

Voiding cystometry

- Permission to void is given.
- The patient empties their bladder with the pressure transducers still in place, enabling correlation of flow with detrusor pressure.
- This assesses for contractility of the detrusor and can elicit use of abdominal straining.

❶ Some women may be inhibited by the situation and the pressure catheters. Voiding dysfunction should therefore not be diagnosed on this test alone—uroflowmetry in privacy may give a truer picture of voiding function.

Additional urodynamic tests

Ambulatory urodynamics

This gives a more 'physiological' approach to cystometry and overcomes some of the issues that occur with a standard test such as non-physiological filling and inhibition.

- Microtip transducers record rectal and bladder pressures.
- The bladder is filled physiologically (i.e. no filling line, patient drinking normally).
- Studies can last for several hours and allow the patient to carry out more life-like tests of provocation.
- Measures of leakage:
  - Patient presses event marker (subjective)
  - Pad weight gain measured over duration of test.

Use

Particularly useful if a conventional test has been unable to reproduce symptoms. It has a higher sensitivity for eliciting detrusor overactivity than a standard test, and helps to differentiate whether leakage is due to detrusor activity or stress incontinence where the diagnosis is unclear.

Videourodynamics (videocystourethrography)

Synchronous radiological screening of the bladder and measurement of the bladder and abdominal pressure during filling and voiding cystometry. The bladder is filled with iodine-based contrast and fluoroscopy allows visualization of bladder 'events' and morphology.

- Detrusor contractions can be seen directly
- Allows observation of position of bladder neck in relation to pubic symphysis
- Looks at bladder neck closure at rest and under stress
- Demonstrates diverticulae
- Looks for vesicoureteric reflux
- Demonstrates detrusor-sphincter-dyssynergia.

❶ It may be particularly useful in the assessment of patients with neurogenic bladder conditions.

Urethral pressure profilometry (UPP)

• Tests of urethral function.

Technique for UPP
• A catheter with a pressure transducer is withdrawn at constant speed from the bladder neck to the urethral meatus.
• This measures the intraluminal pressure along the length of the urethra.

▶ If the squeeze pressure of the urethra is greater than the intravesical pressure, then continence will be maintained.

Use
• UPPs were previously used to determine which continence surgery should be performed for SUI.
• They differentiate incontinence due to sphincter deficiency from that due to hypermobility.
• Traditionally patients with hypermobility were treated with colposuspension whereas those with sphincter deficiency were offered sling procedures.

◐ Urogynaecological practice changed to almost all patients being offered mid-urethral slings, and hence UPP measurement was rarely indicated.

❶ It is an invasive and poorly reproducible test, and as such is usually reserved for research purposes rather than clinical practice.

Lower urinary tract conditions

Overactive bladder syndrome: overview 28
Overactive bladder syndrome: management 30
Stress urinary incontinence: overview 34
Stress urinary incontinence: conservative management 36
Stress urinary incontinence: surgical management 38
SUI: urethral bulking injections 40
SUI: synthetic mid-urethral slings 42
SUI: colposuspension 44
SUI: autologous fascial sling 46
SUI: artificial urinary sphincter 48
Recurrent SUI 50
Other types of urinary incontinence 52
Voiding dysfunction 54
Drugs that affect bladder function 56

Overactive bladder syndrome: overview

Definition
- Urinary urgency, usually accompanied by frequency and nocturia, with or without urgency urinary incontinence, in the absence of urinary tract infection or other obvious pathology.
- Used to imply underlying DO but this diagnosis requires urodynamic testing.

Incidence
- Estimated that 1 in 6 women will be affected
- Increases with age
- Second most common cause of urinary incontinence in women.

Aetiology
- Usually idiopathic
- May be neurogenic, e.g. multiple sclerosis, upper motor neuron lesions (➔ see Chapter 7, Neurology)
- May occur secondary to pelvic floor or incontinence surgery
- Rarely due to outflow obstruction.

History
- Frequency
- Urgency, with or without incontinence
- Nocturia
- Nocturnal enuresis
- Symptoms may be provoked, e.g. by cold, running taps, key in the front door, etc.
- Detrusor contractions may also be provoked by increased abdominal pressure, e.g. coughing, laughing, which can be confused with SUI
- Leakage with orgasm is thought to be secondary to detrusor contraction
- Leakage associated with urgency can be unpredictable and of large volume.

Assessment
- Exclude UTI with dipstick and culture
- Frequency/volume chart—typically shows increased frequency, nocturia, reduced functional bladder capacity
- Urodynamic investigations should be considered if initial management has failed or in complex patients
- Consider other factors contributing to symptoms such as diabetes causing polyuria or faecal impaction
- See Fig. 3.1.

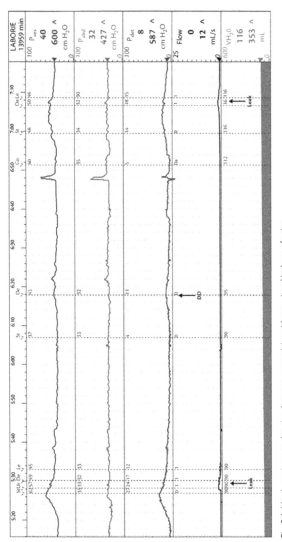

Fig. 3.1 Urodynamic trace showing detrusor overactivity with associated leakage of urine.

Reprinted from Jones and Hashim: Urodynamics, in the *Oxford Textbook of Urological Surgery*, Eds: Hamdy F and Eardley I (2017) Oxford: Oxford University Press, with permission from Oxford University Press

Overactive bladder syndrome: management

Conservative management

▶ All women should be given information about self-help measures and simple lifestyle interventions.

Fluid management
- Aim for 1–1.5L liquids a day (many women may fluid restrict due to how their bladder behaves which may make things worse)
- Avoid caffeine (tea, coffee, chocolate drinks, cola, energy drinks)
- Avoid alcoholic drinks.

Optimize medical conditions
- Review drugs that alter bladder function, e.g. diuretics, antipsychotics
- Optimize glycaemic control if diabetic
- Advise weight loss if BMI >30.

Bladder retraining
- Also termed bladder drill
- Techniques to suppress urgency and extend the interval between voids
- Can be self-taught or assisted by continence advisor or physiotherapist
- Pelvic floor muscle training is of benefit, particularly for those with mixed symptoms.

Supportive management
- Offer input from continence advisor/community continence team.
- Absorbent products (pads/pants) can be used as an adjunct to other management strategies and in some cases, patients may be offered these on prescription or delivery service.
- Home toileting devices or commodes may be beneficial if mobility is reduced.

Pharmacological management

Oestrogen
- Women with vaginal atrophy may benefit from intravaginal oestrogen.
- Systemic HRT should not be used solely for urinary symptoms.

Anticholinergic (antimuscarinic) drugs
- Remain the mainstay of drug treatment of OAB.
- Work by parasympathetic blockade, thus relaxing the detrusor muscle.
- Dosage needs to be titrated against efficacy and side effects (see Table 3.1).
- Side effects of anticholinergic drugs include:
  - dry mouth (up to 30%)
  - GI upset: constipation, nausea, dyspepsia
  - neurological symptoms: insomnia, dizziness, blurred vision.
- Recent evidence shows a link between 'anticholinergic burden' and increased risk of dementia. Patients should be advised that the long-term effects of anticholinergic drugs on cognitive function are uncertain.
- Patients should be advised about the risks and side effects of treatment, and also informed that it may take up to 4 weeks to see the benefits.

Table 3.1 Anticholinergic drugs

Drug	Dose (adult)	Selectivity	Notes
Oxybutynin	2.5–5mg, 2–4 times/day	M1, M3	Use reduced dose in elderly and avoid if frail (risk of falls and confusion) Transdermal patch available (may have reduced side effects)
Tolterodine	2mg twice daily	Non-selective	
Fesoterodine	4–8mg once daily	M3	
Solifenacin	5–10mg once daily	M3	
Darifenacin	7.5–15mg once daily	M3	
Trospium	20mg twice daily	Non-selective	Less likely to cross blood-brain barrier

---

❶ Contraindications to anticholinergic drugs

- Closed angle glaucoma
- Myasthenia gravis
- Urinary retention/outflow obstruction
- Severe ulcerative colitis
- GI obstruction.

β-3 adrenergic agonists (mirabegron)

- Causes relaxation of the detrusor muscle with increased bladder capacity
- Contraindicated in uncontrolled hypertension
- Well tolerated.

Botulinum toxin A

- Blocks neuromuscular transmission, causing weakness of the detrusor
- Injected cystoscopically into the detrusor muscle
- Can be performed under local anaesthesia for the majority of patients and is well tolerated
- High efficacy
- Effect is temporary and lasts 6–12 months so repeat injections are offered if patient satisfied with treatment
- Risk (5–20%) of urinary retention requiring patient to perform CIC until effects wear off. Patients must be counselled regarding this and must be willing to perform CIC if necessary. Patients at increased risk of voiding dysfunction should be taught CIC prior to first treatment.

▶ The long-term effect of repeat injections is still unclear.

Neurostimulation

Percutaneous posterior tibial nerve stimulation
- The exact mechanism of action of PTNS on the bladder is unclear, but it is thought to be mediated by retrograde stimulation of the sacral nerve plexus.
- A fine needle is inserted above the ankle, next to the tibial nerve, and is electrically stimulated.
- Initial treatment is usually 30-min sessions once weekly for 12 weeks.
- It is effective in the short and medium term but effects diminish over time.

Percutaneous sacral nerve stimulation
- Electrode leads are implanted next to sacral nerves and connected to an impulse generator.
- A test wire is inserted first, and if beneficial a permanent implant may be considered.
- May be beneficial but funding in the UK is limited.

Surgery

- Reserved for those with debilitating symptoms who have not responded to other therapies.

Detrusor myectomy
- Detrusor muscle fibres are stripped from the bladder
- Success no better than less invasive treatments such as botulinum toxin.

Augmentation cystoplasty
- Bladder is enlarged using ileum
- High morbidity—metabolic derangement, malignancy developing in ileal segment of neo-bladder.

Urinary diversion

Occasionally indicated in women with intractable incontinence (➔ see Chapter 5, Urology, p. 110; see also NICE Clinical guideline [NG123]. Urinary incontinence and pelvic organ prolapse in women: management. April 2019).

Stress urinary incontinence: overview

Definition
Complaint of involuntary loss of urine on effort or physical exertion including sporting activities, etc., or on sneezing or coughing.

Incidence
- Commonest cause of incontinence in women
- Estimated that 1:10 women will experience SUI (may be underreported)
- May be pure SUI or mixed (coexisting OAB symptoms).

Pathophysiology
- Continence requires urethral pressure to be greater than intravesical pressure
- SUI occurs when intravesical pressure exceeds urethral closing pressure
- Two potential mechanisms that may coexist:
  - Urethral hypermobility (impaired pelvic floor support)
  - Intrinsic sphincter deficiency (denervation or weakness of sphincter mechanism)
- Most frequently seen as a consequence of childbirth
- Oestrogen deficiency leads to weakened pelvic floor support and thinning of the urothelium, hence symptoms frequently deteriorate at menopause.

Risk factors
- Parity
- Menopausal status
- Raised intraabdominal pressure (chronic cough, constipation)
- Obesity
- Pelvic floor denervation (surgery, e.g. hysterectomy, radiotherapy)
- Connective tissue disorders.

History
- Leakage provoked by activity, coughing, laughing, sneezing, penetration, etc.

Assessment
- Examination: atrophy, urethral descent with straining, leakage may be demonstrable with coughing
- Assess pelvic floor muscle contraction
- Urine dipstick and MSU to exclude infection
- Frequency/volume chart: usually shows normal voiding pattern and functional bladder capacity but may show evidence of 'precautionary voiding' (more frequent voids to try and prevent leakage)
- Urodynamic assessment—leakage seen with raised intraabdominal pressure in the absence of a detrusor contraction.

Stress urinary incontinence: conservative management

▶ Conservative measures should always be tried prior to consideration of invasive treatment and in many patients will be sufficient to manage symptoms.

Lifestyle
- Weight loss if BMI >30
- Management of chronic cough or constipation
- Smoking cessation.

Pelvic floor muscle training
- Women should be offered supervised pelvic floor muscle training for a period of 3 months as first-line treatment for SUI.
- Programmes should comprise at least 8 contractions performed 3 times per day.
- This should be continued if training is beneficial.
- Patients who cannot contract their pelvic floor may be offered biofeedback (converts contraction into visual or auditory feedback) or electrical stimulation to aid adherence and motivation.

Continence aids
- Intraurethral and intravaginal inserts are available and may be useful for women who only leak with certain circumstances (e.g. to use for sporting activities).

Pharmacological management
- **Duloxetine** is the only drug licensed for management of SUI.
- It is a SNRI (inhibits the reuptake of serotonin and noradrenaline) and is more commonly used as an antidepressant or for neuropathic pain.
- It enhances urethral striated muscle activity via a centrally mediated pathway.
- Dosage: 40mg twice daily (although may commence at half this and increase to minimize side effects).
- Side effects: nausea, dry mouth, insomnia, GI upset, drowsiness.
- Effect is dose-dependent but side effects frequently limit use.
- May be offered if surgery is declined or patient unsuitable for invasive treatment.

▶ Any medical conditions or drugs that may affect continence should be reviewed.

Stress urinary incontinence: surgical management

Considerations
- Conservative treatment should be tried first.
- Surgery is indicated if conservative measures are insufficient to control symptoms and quality of life is adversely affected.
- It is important to be clear about underlying diagnosis prior to treatment: surgery for SUI may make underlying detrusor overactivity worse. Most would advocate suppressing detrusor overactivity prior to offering treatment for SUI.
- Patients should be advised to defer surgery until childbearing is complete.
- Surgical options will depend on patient factors (obesity, previous surgery, medical comorbidity) and surgeon factors (experience and training).
- All options should be reviewed with the patient, and an individualized assessment of benefit and risk discussed.
- Decision-making should be a collaborative process between patient and clinician.
- If a patient opts for a treatment that is not performed locally a regional referral should be offered.
- All patients should be reviewed and discussed in a multidisciplinary team meeting.

Surgical options
- Periurethral bulking
- Synthetic mid-urethral slings (note: currently 'paused' by NHS England—**ᗒ** see Chapter 11)
- Colposuspension—open or laparoscopic
- Autologous fascial sling
- Artificial urinary sphincter.

---

❶ The following should not be offered to treat SUI:
- Anterior colporrhaphy
- Needle suspensions
- Marshall–Marchetti–Krantz procedures
- Paravaginal defect repairs.

Resources
ᗒ NICE Clinical guideline [NG123]. Urinary incontinence and pelvic organ prolapse in women: management. April 2019.

SUI: urethral bulking injections

Technique
- Injections around the urethra to create urethral cushions, improving coaptation and therefore improving continence.
- The ideal bulking agent should be non-immunogenic, hypoallergenic, deformable, and durable.
- Various materials have been used including collagen, water-based gels, silicone, and carbon-coated zirconium beads.
- There is insufficient evidence to guide whether efficacy is greater when injected at the bladder neck or at the mid-urethra.
- Treatment is injected via a cystoscope and may be performed under local or general anaesthesia.

Advantages
- Minimally invasive
- Low morbidity
- Doesn't preclude further continence surgery if unsuccessful
- May be suitable for women who are frail, have comorbidities, or who have not completed their family.

Disadvantages
- Repeat injections may be needed to achieve efficacy
- Effect diminishes over time
- Lower success compared to more invasive procedures.

Outcomes
- 60% will report improvement in symptoms, although effects diminish with time and many women will request further injection or an alternative continence procedure.

Risks of bulking injections
- Haematuria (transient)
- Dysuria (transient)
- Infection
- Voiding difficulty (rare)
- Migration of bulking agent (only seen with particulate agents)
- Abscess formation at bulking site (rare).

SUI: synthetic mid-urethral slings

🚫 Vaginally inserted mesh is currently 'paused' by NHS England

Technique—general principles

- Synthetic material (polypropylene) placed at the level of the mid-urethra to create support (see Fig. 3.2).
- Approach may be retropubic or transobturator.
- It is recommended that coloured mesh is used for ease of insertion and revision.
- Implants should be considered permanent and patients counselled accordingly.

➔ See Chapter 11, Miscellaneous, p. 172 for further discussion about the use of mesh.

Retropubic approach

- Up until the recent 'pause' of mesh procedures, TVT was the most commonly performed procedure for SUI in the UK.
- The 'bottom-up' technique is most commonly used. A 'top-down' approach should only be used in the context of research.
- A small vaginal incision is made at the level of the mid-urethra.
- Dissection is used laterally to create tunnels.
- The introducers are passed from the vaginal entry point through the retropubic space and exit suprapubically.
- A cystoscopy is performed to exclude bladder perforation.
- The tape is adjusted and left loose (tension free).

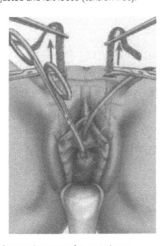

Fig. 3.2 Insertion of retropubic tension-free vaginal tape.
Illustration reproduced by courtesy of ETHICON Women's Health and Urology

Transobturator approach
- The tape is passed from the vaginal incision via the transobturator foramen, passing through obturator membrane and adductor muscles, exiting through small incisions in the groin.
- There is less long-term outcome data for this approach compared to TVT.
- There is a higher incidence of chronic buttock or groin pain following this technique.
- This approach should be reserved for patients with whom avoiding the retropubic space is advised (e.g. previous pelvic surgery).

Advantages
- High efficacy
- Day case procedures.

Disadvantages
- Use of mesh is highly controversial at present
- Risk of mesh complications
- Risk of voiding dysfunction
- Risk of new or worsening urgency.

Outcomes
- Objective cure rate 80–90%.

Risks of mid-urethral slings
- Generic surgical risks (bleeding, infection, anaesthetic risk, DVT, visceral or vascular injury).
- Intraoperative bladder injury: common. This should be recognized at the check cystoscopy and the tape repositioned. It is not known to have any long-term sequelae.
- Worsening of or de novo urgency.
- Voiding difficulties. This may be temporary but can persist (approximately 5%). The tape can be loosened up to 14 days following surgery (the longer post-surgery, the less likely this is to be technically possible as fibrosis occurs).
- Chronic pain—pelvic, vaginal, and groin pain have all been reported. This is more common with the transobturator approach.
- Mesh exposure in the vagina which may require revision surgery.
- Mesh exposure in the bladder or urethra (this may represent a missed injury at the time of surgery, or a de novo erosion). Usually requires mesh removal.
- ⊃ See Chapter 11, Miscellaneous, p. 172 for more information about use and complications of mesh.

SUI: colposuspension

Burch (open) colposuspension
- Considered gold standard prior to the introduction of TVT.
- The retropubic space is accessed via a low transverse suprapubic incision.
- 2–3 sutures are placed between the paravaginal fascia and ipsilateral iliopectineal (Cooper's) ligament on each side, elevating the bladder neck.
- Sutures may be permanent or absorbable depending on surgeon and patient preference.
- This technique requires mobility of the anterior vaginal wall, and so may be unsuitable if the vaginal wall is scarred from previous surgery or very atrophic and immobile.

Laparoscopic colposuspension
- Requires considerable laparoscopic expertise
- Approach may be intraabdominal or extraperitoneal
- Outcome data is predominantly extrapolated from studies of open colposuspension.

Advantages
- Treats cystocoele in addition to SUI
- High efficacy.

Disadvantages
- Longer recovery than a TVT
- Risk of voiding dysfunction
- Risk of worsening or de novo urgency
- Risk of developing posterior compartment prolapse.

Outcomes
- Objective cure rate 80–90%
- May diminish over time (cure rate 70% at 20y).

Risks of colposuspension
- Generic surgical risks (bleeding, infection, anaesthetic risk, DVT, wound complications, visceral or vascular injury)
- Worsening of or de novo urgency (up to 17%)
- Voiding difficulties (up to 10%)
- Posterior compartment prolapse (up to 14%)
- Dyspareunia
- Suture erosion (with non-absorbable sutures)—into vagina or bladder.

SUI: autologous fascial sling

Technique

- A strip of rectus fascia is harvested via a lower transverse suprapubic abdominal incision.
- This is then used to create a sling around the urethra.
- Different techniques have been described to insert the fascia:
  - The traditional 'Aldridge sling' describes a top-down approach, maintaining medial attachment of two fascial strips and passing the lateral portions retropubically into a vaginal incision, where the strips are then sutured in the midline at the bladder neck.
  - The newer 'sling on a string' technique harvests one smaller strip of fascia and inserts using the same technique as for a retropubic tape.
- Other techniques describe using fascia lata rather than rectus fascia.

Advantages

- This appeals to patients who wish to avoid use of mesh
- Success rates are similar to TVT.

Disadvantages

- Longer recovery due to abdominal wound
- Risk of incisional hernia
- Higher risk of voiding dysfunction compared to other procedures
- Risk of worsening or de novo urgency.

Outcomes

- Objective cure rate 80–90%.

Risks of fascial slings

- Generic surgical risks (bleeding, infection, anaesthetic risk, DVT, wound complications, visceral or vascular injury)
- Worsening of or de novo urgency (up to 10%)
- Voiding difficulties (up to 10%)
- Hernia formation (up to 10%)
- Dyspareunia.

SUI: artificial urinary sphincter

Technique

▶ This is usually reserved for patients who have failed other surgical approaches for SUI.
- A circular cuff is inserted around the urethra to maintain closure.
- This is controlled via a pump inserted under the skin of the labia majora which operates a fluid filled reservoir inserted in the subrectus space.

Advantages

- Mimics physiological continence mechanism.

Disadvantages

- Invasive procedure with significant morbidity
- Devices have a limited lifespan (typically 7–10y)
- Risk of device being explanted due to infection or migration.

Outcomes

- 70% of women are completely dry, with 90% happy overall with the results.

Risks of artificial sphincters

- Generic surgical risks (bleeding, infection, anaesthetic risk, DVT, wound complications, visceral or vascular injury)
- Voiding difficulties (up to 10%)
- Worsening of or de novo urgency (up to 10%)
- Device issues: infection requiring device removal (up to 10%), device failure (up to 10%), migration into urethra/vagina/abdominal wall (up to 2%).

Recurrent SUI

▶ If initial surgical treatment of SUI has failed, or if symptoms recur after initial successful treatment, patients should be referred to a tertiary centre for assessment.

Assessment

- Urodynamic assessment is required to assess for detrusor overactivity and voiding function in addition to confirming recurrent urodynamic stress incontinence.
- Look for the presence of any complications of the primary surgery.

Management

- Will depend on patient desire for treatment, medical and surgical comorbidity, patient and surgeon preference.
- Repeat surgery will increase the risk of subsequent voiding dysfunction.

Other types of urinary incontinence

Mixed incontinence
- Where SUI and OAB coexist.
- When assessing the patient, it is important to establish which is the most bothersome symptom.
- It can be difficult to distinguish between SUI and provoked DO without urodynamic testing.
- Invasive treatments for SUI are likely to aggravate DO. Most clinicians therefore advocate suppressing DO prior to embarking on surgical treatment of SUI.

Overflow incontinence
- Results from outflow obstruction (stricture, detrusor-sphincter-dyssynergia) or acontractility of the detrusor muscle. Outflow obstruction is rare in females.
- Symptoms include frequency, nocturia, hesitancy, poor stream, straining, revisiting, and recurrent UTI.
- Treatment options include removing the cause of obstruction, behavioural measures such as timed voiding and double voiding, and catheters (intermittent or indwelling).

Functional incontinence
- Mental or physical problems stop the patient from getting to the toilet on time, resulting in leakage.
- Causes include dementia, arthritis, and poor mobility.
- Frequently an issue for the elderly or frail patient.

Ectopic ureter
- Ureter inserts at a site other than the bladder neck such as the urethra, vestibule, or vagina.
- 80% associated with duplex collecting system.
- Typically present in childhood with continuous dribbling of urine after the age of toilet training, recurrent UTI, or watery vaginal discharge.
- Diagnosis is on CT urogram.
- Treatment is surgical.

Voiding dysfunction

Definition
- Abnormally slow and/or incomplete micturition
- Diagnosed from symptoms and urodynamic investigations.

Acute urinary retention
- Inability to pass any urine, with a painful, palpable/percussable bladder.

Chronic urinary retention
- Chronic high postvoid residual measurements.

Symptoms of voiding dysfunction
- Hesitancy
- Slow stream
- Straining
- Feeling of incomplete emptying
- Revisiting shortly after voiding
- Micturition may be positional (e.g. needing to rock forward to initiate or complete a void)
- Frequency, urgency, nocturia
- UTI
- Incontinence.

Causes
- Ageing ($\downarrow$detrusor contractility and $\uparrow$urethral rigidity)
- Constipation
- Postsurgery
- Postpartum
- Neurological disease (detrusor sphincter dyssynergia)
- Psychological (the 'bashful bladder')
- Severe pelvic organ prolapse
- Overdistension of the bladder
- Medications (anaesthetic, analgesics, anticholinergics, antidepressants, antipsychotics, botulinum toxin)
- Pelvic mass
- Urethral pathology
- Vulval skin conditions (e.g. lichen sclerosus casing fusion).

Assessment
- Look for underlying cause
- Uroflowmetry
- Measurement of postvoid residual
- Cystometry.

Management

- Treat underlying cause if possible, e.g. treat prolapse, remove pelvic mass, loosen sling
- Aid bladder emptying—intermittent self-catheterization or indwelling catheters
- If detrusor under-contractility is present, the patient may benefit from nerve stimulation, e.g. PTNS or SNS.

Fowler's syndrome

- A cause of urinary retention in young women.
- Due to failure of relaxation of the urethral sphincter.
- The underlying cause is unknown.
- An association with PCOS has been reported.
- The onset may be spontaneous, or may follow childbirth or an unrelated operative procedure.
- Symptoms include those of poor emptying, recurrent UTI, and sometimes acute retention.
- The gold standard for diagnosis is a sphincter EMG.
- Treatment is with intermittent self-catheterization (although this can be painful and may not be possible in patients with Fowler's), indwelling catheters, or SNS.

Drugs that affect bladder function

- Drugs with anticholinergic properties (antidepressants, antipsychotics)—can cause retention and potentially overflow.
- α-blockers (used as antihypertensives)—urethral relaxation resulting in stress incontinence.
- Diuretics—increase urine output, resulting in polyuria, frequency, nocturia.
- Calcium channel blockers—decrease detrusor contractility resulting in retention and potentially overflow.
- Sedatives/hypnotics—may lead to functional incontinence.
- ACE inhibitors—diuretic effect, plus cough is a common side effect and may exacerbate stress incontinence.

Pelvic organ prolapse

Overview 58
Grading of pelvic organ prolapse 60
Assessment 62
Management: conservative 64
Management: pessaries 66
Management: principles of surgery 68
Surgery for cystocele 70
Surgery for enterocele/rectocele 72
Surgery for uterine prolapse 74
Surgery for vaginal vault prolapse 78
Surgery: obliterative procedures 80
Recurrent prolapse 82

Overview

Definition
POP is where the pelvic organs (uterus/vaginal apex/bladder/bowel) herniate into or beyond the vagina from their normal anatomical position.

Prevalence
▶ The true prevalence of POP is unknown, as many women are asymptomatic or do not seek medical attention.
- It is estimated that half of all parous women have some loss of pelvic floor support, and that of these 10–20% will seek help.
- The lifetime risk of undergoing pelvic floor surgery by the age of 80 is 11%.

Aetiology
- *Parity and childbirth*. POP is uncommon in nulliparous women. The risk of developing POP increases with increasing parity, larger babies, instrumental birth (forceps > ventouse), and prolonged second stage.
  - Direct injury and denervation weaken the pelvic floor.
  - Perineal injury may widen the genital hiatus.
- *Connective tissue*. There is an association between POP and hypermobility conditions, e.g. Ehlers–Danlos syndrome.
- *Ageing and the menopause*. There is a deterioration in the quantity and quality of collagen in connective tissue in older, postmenopausal women. It is difficult to separate the effect of age and of oestrogen deficiency.
- *Increased intraabdominal pressure*. For example, chronic cough, constipation, increased BMI, prolonged heavy lifting, pelvic mass.
- *Congenital*. Some congenital conditions have an increased incidence of POP, e.g. bladder exstrophy is commonly associated with POP.
- *Pelvic surgery*.
  - Hysterectomy divides the uterosacral and cardinal ligaments and so may predispose to prolapse formation. This risk increases if the hysterectomy was performed for prolapse.
  - Colposuspension (bladder neck elevation) predisposes to recto-enterocoele formation.
  - Sacrospinous ligament fixation may predispose to anterior compartment prolapse.
- *Ethnic origin*. POP is rare in women of African/East Asian descent.

Classification of POP

Prolapse is classified anatomically according to the site of the defect and the pelvic organs involved (Fig. 4.1).

- *Cystocele*—prolapse of the anterior vaginal wall, involving the bladder. If there is coexisting urethral prolapse, the term cystourethrocele is used.
- *Apical prolapse*—prolapse of the uterus, cervix, and upper vagina, or of the vaginal vault if the uterus is absent.
- *Enterocele*—prolapse of the upper posterior vaginal wall, usually containing loops of small bowel.
- *Rectocele*—prolapse of the lower posterior vaginal wall involving the rectum.

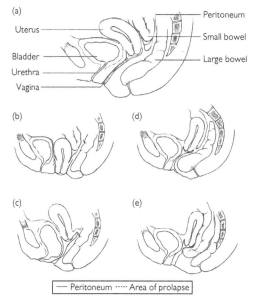

Fig. 4.1 Types of prolapse. (a) Normal pelvis, (b) uterine prolapse, (c) cystocele, (d) rectocele, (e) enterocele.

Reprinted from Impey L and Child T (2012) *Obstetrics and Gynaecology*. Oxford: Wiley-Blackwell publishing, with permission from John Wiley & Sons

Grading of pelvic organ prolapse

- Several grading systems have been used to describe pelvic organ prolapse.
- The two most commonly in use are the Baden–Walker classification and the POP-Q scoring system.

Baden–Walker classification of prolapse

- *First degree*—the lowest part of the prolapse descends halfway down the vaginal axis towards the introitus.
- *Second degree*—the lowest part of the prolapse descends to the level of the introitus.
- *Third degree*—the lowest part of the prolapse descends through the introitus and lies outside the vagina (also called procidentia).

POP-Q system

- This aims to standardize the description of POP, providing a more objective and reproducible assessment.
- Nine points in the vagina are measured in reference to the hymen, in the left lateral position at rest, and at Valsalva.
- See Tables 4.1 and 4.2, and Fig. 4.2.

Table 4.1 Landmarks for POP-Q (ranges in brackets)

Aa	Anterior vaginal wall 3 cm proximal to the hymen (−3cm to +3cm)
Ba	Most distal position of the remaining upper anterior vaginal wall (−3cm to +tvl)
C	Most distal edge of cervix or vaginal cuff scar
D	Posterior fornix (N/A if posthysterectomy)
Ap	Posterior vaginal wall 3cm proximal to the hymen (−3cm to +3cm)
Bp	Most distal position of the remaining upper posterior vaginal wall (−3cm to + tvl)
Genital hiatus (gh)	Measured from middle of external urethral meatus to posterior midline hymen
Perineal body (bp)	Measured from posterior margin of gh to middle of anal opening
Total vaginal length (tvl)	Depth of vagina when point D or C is reduced to normal position

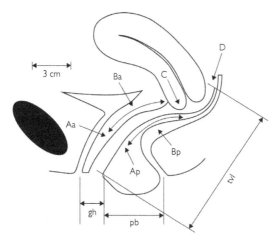

Fig. 4.2 Points and landmarks for POP-Q system examination (see Table 4.1 for further details).

Reprinted from Bump RC et al (1996) 'The standardization of terminology of female pelvic organ prolapse and pelvic floor dysfunction' Am J Obstet Gynecol. 175(1):10–17 with permission from Elsevier

Table 4.2 POP-Q staging

Stage	Description
0	No prolapse
1	Most distal portion of the prolapse is more than 1cm above the level of the hymen
2	Most distal portion of the prolapse is 1 cm or less proximal to or distal to the plane of the hymen
3	Most distal portion of the prolapse is more than 1cm below the plane of the hymen
4	Complete eversion of the total length of the lower genital tract (procidentia)

Source: data from Persu C et al (2011) 'Pelvic Organ Prolapse Quantification System (POP–Q)— a new era in pelvic prolapse staging' J. Med Life 4(1):75–81.

Assessment

Symptoms
🛈 There is often surprisingly little correlation between severity of symptoms and examination findings.

Vaginal symptoms
- Heaviness, dragging sensation
- 'Something coming down'
- A lump that may be seen outside the vagina and may need digital replacement
- Difficulty retaining tampons
- Sexual dysfunction
- May cause friction, ulceration, and bleeding if prolapse descends past the introitus.

Bladder symptoms (anterior compartment prolapse)
- Urgency, frequency
- Incomplete emptying
- Need to change position to void
- Recurrent UTI (if significant postvoid residual)
- Ureteric obstruction/hydronephrosis in severe procidentia (rare).

Bowel symptoms (posterior compartment prolapse)
- Difficulty in emptying
- Need to digitate vagina or splint perineum to empty.

▶ Backache can be associated with prolapse but is difficult to differentiate from other common causes of lower back pain.

Quality of life
Treatment should be based on symptoms and impact on quality of life. Validated assessment tools such as the ICIQ-VS may help evaluate this.

Examination
- Look for atrophy, ulceration.
- Bimanual to exclude pelvic mass.
- Assess and grade the prolapse: in left lateral position, using a Sims's speculum, each vaginal wall and the apex are inspected and the patient asked to bear down.
- Sometimes a prolapse will only be demonstrated in the standing position.
- Grade pelvic floor muscle strength (see Table 4.3).

▶ Further investigations are rarely required.

Table 4.3 Modified Oxford system for grading pelvic floor muscle strength

A system of grading using vaginal palpation of the pelvic floor muscles.	
0	No contraction
1	Flicker
2	Weak
3	Moderate
4	Good (with lift)
5	Strong

Management: conservative

When to consider conservative management:
- Asymptomatic prolapse
- If the patient has not yet completed her family and can defer definitive treatment
- If the patient is unfit for invasive treatment
- If this is the patient's wish.

▶ Patients should be reassured that prolapse is a benign condition and that the only indication for treatment is patient desire.

Lifestyle measures
- Weight loss
- Manage constipation
- Treatment of chronic cough (including smoking cessation).

Oestrogen
- Vaginal oestrogen will not fix the mechanical problem but may relieve symptoms of itchiness and dryness and help resolve ulceration.

Physiotherapy
- Pelvic floor muscle training can reduce symptoms and limit progression of milder prolapse.

Management: pessaries

These are vinyl or silicon devices of varying sizes and shapes that support the vagina and/or uterus.

Indications for pessary
- Patient preference
- As a short-term measure while waiting for surgery
- For prolapse that occurs during pregnancy.

Pessary fitting
- Digital examination is used to estimate vaginal size.
- A successful pessary should be comfortable and adequately control the prolapse.
- Start small and increase in size as needed.
- If the pessary is too small it is unlikely to be retained or may not control the prolapse.
- If it is too large it will be uncomfortable.
- Patients should be warned that it can be trial and error finding the correct pessary for them.

Ongoing management
- Pessaries should be changed every 6 months as a minimum (more frequently for shelf/Gellhorn types).
- Use of vaginal oestrogen is recommended to reduce the risk of excoriation.

Issues with pessaries
- Retention
- Discharge (common)
- Ulceration and bleeding
- Vaginal bands resulting in difficult changes
- Fistula (rare—seen with neglected pessaries).

Pessaries and sexual function
▶ It is vital to establish a patient's desire to continue having intercourse prior to fitting a pessary.
- Intercourse is possible with a ring pessary in situ.
- Patients can be taught to remove and reinsert ring pessaries to facilitate intercourse.
- Intercourse is not possible with shelf or Gellhorn pessaries.

Management: principles of surgery

There are a wide variety of options for surgical management of POP but the underlying principles apply to all.

Principles of surgery

- The ideal operation for POP would relieve symptoms, be long-lasting, have low morbidity, and would preserve sexual function.
- The need for repeat surgery is unfortunately relatively frequent.
- Prolapse is often not isolated to one compartment. In multicompartment prolapse, failure to treat all defects may result in ongoing symptoms.
- Careful management of patient expectation is required, particularly as regards sexual, bladder, and bowel function following surgery.
- Treating prolapse is known to reveal occult SUI in a proportion of cases and patients must be counselled accordingly. There has been a trend to perform concomitant procedures for SUI to prevent this, but this will result in overtreatment and higher morbidity. Most would advocate a more conservative approach and assess for urinary symptoms after correcting POP.
- Surgical preference will depend on training and expertise.
- Patients should be offered choice of treatments, and if a surgeon does not personally perform a particular surgery, the patient should be offered a referral elsewhere if desired. The Urogynaecology community is heading towards regional networks, with close working between secondary and tertiary referral centres.
- A multidisciplinary approach should be the cornerstone of management, with all complex patients, repeat surgeries and mesh implants being discussed and approved within the MDT.

Surgery for cystocele

Anterior colporrhaphy
• May be performed under local, regional, or general anaesthesia
• Low morbidity
• High recurrence (estimated at 30%)—may be in part due to failure to recognize and correct an apical defect.

Technique for anterior colporrhaphy
• Local anaesthetic and adrenaline is infiltrated (for analgesia, vasoconstriction and hydro-dissection). A longitudinal vaginal incision is made and the skin separated from the bladder. The pubocervical fascia is plicated, excess vaginal skin is trimmed and the vagina closed.

Mesh repair
• Numerous mesh kits for augmenting the anterior vaginal wall have been marketed.
• NICE suggests that mesh repairs may be undertaken in the context of research studies.

❶ Vaginal mesh insertion has been suspended at the time of writing.
• ➲ See Chapter 11, Miscellaneous, p. 172 for more on the use of mesh.

Paravaginal repair
• No longer in common use
• This uses an abdominal (or laparoscopic) approach to correct an anterior wall prolapse.

Technique for paravaginal repair
The retropubic space is opened and the bladder swept medially. The lateral vaginal sulci are reattached to the pelvic sidewall.

Sacrocolpopexy
• This technique may be useful for patients following hysterectomy who have recurrent anterior wall prolapse or where there is a concurrent apical defect.
• ➲ See Surgery for vault prolapse, p. 78.

Surgery for enterocele/rectocele

Posterior colporrhaphy

- Performed under regional or general anaesthesia
- Higher morbidity than anterior colporrhaphy (largely relates to postoperative pain, constipation, and vaginal infection)
- Outcomes generally good
- Care must be taken not to excise too much skin as this will shorten and narrow the vagina and can impact on sexual function
- This can also be performed transanally by colorectal surgeons, but outcomes are thought to be better with a vaginal approach.

Technique for posterior colporrhaphy

Local anaesthetic and adrenaline are infiltrated. A longitudinal vaginal wall incision is made, and the rectum is reflected from the vaginal skin. Sutures are used to plicate the rectovaginal fascia. Excess skin is trimmed and the vaginal wall is closed. A rectal examination must be performed to ensure no sutures have passed through the rectum which could result in fistula formation.

This may be combined with a perineorrhaphy (placing deeper sutures into the perineal muscles) to provide additional support.

Mesh repair

- ➜ See previous page (p. 70).

Sacrocolpopexy

- This may be used to correct large enterocele in patients with or without a uterus.

Surgery for uterine prolapse

Vaginal hysterectomy
- The most commonly performed procedure for uterine prolapse.
- Performed under regional or general anaesthesia.
- Usually combined with anterior and/or posterior colporrhaphy.
- This is particularly useful to manage coexisting prolapse and menorrhagia.
- Simply removing the uterus does not support the vaginal vault and so additional steps to support this are usually required.

Technique for vaginal hysterectomy
Local anaesthetic and adrenaline are infiltrated. A circumferential incision is made around the cervix and the bladder is reflected, enabling the operator to access and open the vesicouterine fold. The pouch of Douglas is opened. A series of pedicles are then clamped, divided, and tied; the uterosacral ligaments, the uterine arteries, and the tubo-ovarian and round ligaments, thus separating the uterus from its attachments. After removing the uterus and checking for haemostasis the vaginal vault is closed, and a vaginal wall repair performed if necessary.

The following options are used to create additional vault support:
- *McCall culdoplasty*—the uterosacral ligaments are approximated with a continuous suture to obliterate the peritoneum of the posterior cul-de-sac as high as possible.
- *Uterosacral ligament suspension*—the uterosacral pedicles are sutured to the vaginal vault.
- *Sacrospinous ligament fixation*—if the vaginal vault descends to the level of the introitus when closing, this should be considered.

Manchester repair
- Performed under regional or general anaesthesia
- This combines amputation of the cervix with a vaginal repair
- This technique may of benefit for women with cervical elongation.

Technique for Manchester repair
Local anaesthetic and adrenaline are infiltrated. The initial steps are as for vaginal hysterectomy. A circumferential incision is made around the cervix and the bladder is reflected. The vesicouterine fold is opened, as is the pouch of Douglas. The uterosacral ligaments are clamped, divided, and tied. The cervix is then amputated, and the uterosacral ligaments are sutured to the lower uterine segment. Anterior and/or posterior repair is undertaken, then the vaginal mucosa is closed, ensuring a drainage point is left in the uterine canal for secretions.

Sacrospinous (vaginal) hysteropexy

- Performed under regional or general anaesthesia
- Outcomes are reported to be comparable to vaginal hysterectomy
- Often combined with anterior/posterior colporrhaphy.

Technique for sacrospinous hysteropexy

- Local anaesthetic and adrenaline are infiltrated. The posterior wall is opened up to the posterior part of the cervix. Blunt and sharp dissection is used to visualize the right sacrospinous ligament. Non-absorbable sutures are placed through the sacrospinous ligament and through the posterior aspect of the cervix. Additional vaginal wall repair may be undertaken as needed.

Abdominal hysteropexy

- This is now usually performed laparoscopically, although may be open.
- Requires general anaesthetic.
- Offers the option of uterine preservation if fertility is desired.
- The theoretical advantage is stronger apical support as compared to hysterectomy, but long-term data is currently lacking.
- Correcting the apical defect is likely to resolve vaginal wall prolapse but additional vaginal repair may be offered as required.
- See Fig. 4.3.

Technique for abdominal hysteropexy

The peritoneum over the sacral promontory is opened to expose a safe periosteal window for fixation. The peritoneum is opened from here into the pouch of Douglas, leaving the ureter lateral. The bladder is reflected and bilateral windows made in the broad ligament. A bifurcated polypropylene mesh is inserted, the arms are brought through the windows and sutured to the cervix anteriorly. The mesh is attached to the sacral promontory using a helical fastener. The peritoneum is closed over the mesh to bury it completely.

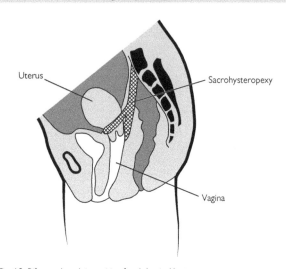

Fig. 4.3 Bifurcated mesh in position for abdominal hysteropexy.

Reprinted from Leron E and Stanton S (2003) 'Sacrohysteropexy with synthetic mesh for the management of uterovaginal prolapse' *BJOG: An International Journal of Obstetrics & Gynaecology* 108(6):629–33 with permission from John Wiley & Sons

Surgery for vaginal vault prolapse

▶ The incidence of posthysterectomy vaginal vault prolapse is estimated at 11.6% when the original hysterectomy was performed for prolapse.

Sacrospinous ligament fixation (SSF)

- This approaches the issue vaginally and is usually combined with posterior and/or anterior colporrhaphy.
- May be performed under regional or general anaesthesia.
- Not suitable if there is inadequate vaginal length.

Technique for SSF

Local anaesthetic and adrenaline are infiltrated. The posterior vaginal wall is opened and the rectovaginal space is opened to identify the sacrospinous ligament. Sutures are placed through the ligament, 2cm medial to the ischial spine to avoid the pudendal nerve and vessels. These are fixed to the vaginal vault to suspend it to the ligament. A concomitant posterior and/or anterior vaginal wall repair is usually performed.

Sacrocolpopexy

- Originally this was described as an open procedure (ASC) but now is frequently performed laparoscopically (LSC).
- Requires general anaesthesia.
- A polypropylene mesh is used over the apex and anterior and posterior vaginal walls and attached to the sacral promontory.
  Several trials have compared ASC with SSF:
- Patients may recover quicker from SSF as compared to abdominal sacrocolpopexy.
- Higher rates of sexual dysfunction are reported with SSF as compared to ASC, as the vaginal axis is changed.
- ASC has a lower long-term risk of recurrent vaginal vault prolapse.
- ASC and LSC are equally effective. LSC has the advantages of minimal access surgery but requires advanced laparoscopic skills.

Technique for sacrocolpopexy

The peritoneum over the sacral promontory is opened and a safe periosteal window for fixation is identified. The peritoneum is opened from here into the pouch of Douglas. The bladder and rectum are reflected from the vaginal vault (a Deaver retractor in the vagina helps to define the anatomy). A Y-shaped polypropylene mesh is sutured to the anterior and posterior vaginal walls. The tail of the mesh is fixed to the sacral promontory with helical fasteners or sutures, and the peritoneum closed to bury the mesh.

Resources

⮀ Post-Hysterectomy Vaginal Vault Prolapse (RCOG Green-top Guideline No. 46, 2015).

Surgery: obliterative procedures

Colpocleisis

• Vaginal closure—can be performed in patients with or without a uterus
• Can be performed under local, regional, or general anaesthesia
• May be an option for frail/comorbid patients in whom sexual function is not desired
• Has high rates of postoperative stress urinary incontinence; concomitant mid-urethral slings have been a popular technique to avoid this.

Technique for colpocleisis

• Local anaesthetic and adrenaline are infiltrated. A rectangular strip of mucosa is carefully dissected and excised from the anterior and posterior vaginal walls, which are then apposed and sutured together, leaving drainage channels for secretions. This effectively obliterates the vaginal space.

Recurrent prolapse

- Prolapse surgery often relies on inherently weak connective tissue, and it is unsurprising that recurrence rates are high.
- Patients who present with recurrent prolapse are more likely to have concurrent bladder, bowel, or sexual dysfunction which may make management more challenging.
▶ Recurrent prolapse may be classified as *same site* or *new site*.

Considerations for management

- Need for intervention should be based on patient symptoms and impact on quality of life.
- Options include doing nothing, physiotherapy, pessaries, or surgery.
- NICE guidance recommends that same site recurrence is reviewed via a regional MDT.
- Repeat surgery is often more technically challenging; the tissue tends to be scarred, and with repeat vaginal surgery there is a significant risk of causing vaginal shortening and/or narrowing, resulting in sexual dysfunction.

Urology

Investigations 84
Ureteric stenting 86
Haematuria 88
Urinary tract infection 90
Recurrent UTI 92
Non-bacterial cystitis 94
Bladder pain syndrome 96
Management of bladder pain syndrome 98
Urethral conditions 100
Urinary tract injuries 102
Vesicovaginal fistula 106
Urinary catheters 108
Urinary diversion 110

Investigations

Plain abdominal X-ray
- Assess for stones.

Ultrasound
- Assess renal tract and bladder
- A full bladder helps to identify intravesical or pelvic lesions
- Identify dilatation of upper tracts
- Identify cortical scarring
- Poor for identification of stones
- Can be used to assess postvoid residual.

CT
- Investigation of choice for stones and renal masses
- Can visualize urothelium in suspected bladder masses
- Useful for detection of injury.

Voiding (micturating) cystourethrogram
- Retrograde contrast filling of bladder with serial X-rays performed during voiding
- Use: diagnosis of vesicoureteric reflux, assess for strictures, suspected obstruction, investigation of recurrent UTI in children
- See Fig. 5.1.

Intravenous urography
- IV contrast injected followed by serial X-rays (see Fig. 5.2)
- Has been largely replaced by CT.

Isotope renography
- IV technetium (Tc-99m) with measurement of distribution using a gamma camera
- Static: Tc-99m DMSA injected, imaging at interval. Useful for renal morphology and assessment of scarring
- Dynamic: Tc-99m MAG3 injected with serial imaging. Used to estimate differential of renal function (i.e. are both kidneys contributing equally to renal clearance).

Retrograde ureteropyelogram
- Contrast injected via bladder then imaged via fluoroscopy/ radiography
- Used in ureteric stenting and to identify intraoperative injury of the ureter.

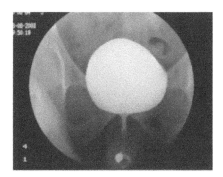

Fig. 5.1 Normal cystogram.
Reprinted from Reynard et al (2019) *Oxford Handbook of Urology* 4th Edition Oxford: Oxford University Press, with permission from Oxford University Press

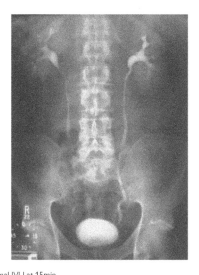

Fig. 5.2 Normal IVU at 15min.
Reprinted from Reynard et al (2019) *Oxford Handbook of Urology* 4th Edition Oxford: Oxford University Press, with permission from Oxford University Press

Ureteric stenting

▶ Used to re-establish or maintain the patency of the ureter.

Indications
- To relieve obstruction, e.g. stricture, stone, tumour
- To allow healing after ureteric injury/repair/surgery
- Prophylactic insertion if anticipating difficult surgery, e.g. severe endometriosis, pelvic cancer.

Technique for stenting
- Appropriate anaesthesia
- Cystoscopic approach
- Ureters cannulated with guidewire under fluoroscopic guidance
- Stent pushed over guidewire and guidewire removed
- Can be removed under local anaesthesia with flexible cystoscope and grasper.

Complications of stents
- UTI
- Haematuria
- Lower urinary tract symptoms, e.g. frequency, urgency, nocturia
- Pain
- Migration
- Blockage.

Haematuria

• Classified as *visible* (macroscopic or gross haematuria) or *non-visible* (microscopic/dipstick haematuria).

❶ Visible haematuria—20–25% will have underlying malignancy.
❶ Non-visible haematuria—5–10% will have underlying malignancy.

Causes of haematuria
• Infection
• Inflammation (non-bacterial cystitis)
• Malignancy (bladder, ureteric, renal)
• Stones
• Trauma
• Renal cysts
• Anticoagulation
• Exercise induced (transient)
• Renal disease: IgA nephropathy, glomerulonephritis, vasculitis.

Who to investigate?
• All visible haematuria
• Non-visible haematuria with LUTS after UTI excluded
• Persistent asymptomatic non-visible haematuria.

Investigations
• MSU
• Urine cytology
• Cystoscopy/biopsy
• CT.

Urinary tract infection

Definition

- Inflammation of the urinary tract due to microbial invasion.
- Classified as simple (no complicating factors) or complicated (associated functional or anatomical abnormality that increases the risk of treatment failure, e.g. pregnancy, calculi, diabetes, presence of catheter).
- Traditionally a cut off of $>10^5$ colony forming units/ml has been used for diagnosis but recent data suggests this may miss a significant number of symptomatic infections.

Responsible organisms

- *Escherichia coli* (at least 70%)
- *Enterococcus*
- *Klebsiella*
- *Staphylococcus saprophyticus*
- *Proteus*
- *Ureaplasma*.

Presentation

- Acute cystitis (pain, dysuria, frequency, haematuria)
- Pyelonephritis
- Sepsis
- Confusion in older people
- May be asymptomatic or non-specific symptoms such as malaise.

Investigation

- Urinalysis, culture, and sensitivity.

Treatment

- Supportive—increase fluid, analgesia, encourage regular voiding
- Antimicrobial treatment according to local protocols.

▶ In cases of catheter-associated infection, treatment should be started based on symptoms and signs rather than positive results as patients will frequently be colonized.

Resources

European Association of Urology guideline: Urological Infections. ℛ https://uroweb.org/guideline/urological-infections

Recurrent UTI

≥ 3 laboratory-confirmed incidences of UTI in a year. May represent re-infection or relapse.

Risk factors for recurrent UTI
- Vaginal flora:
  - Lactobacilli maintain acidic pH and interfere with bacterial adherence and colonization
  - Postmenopausal loss of oestrogen alters this balance increasing the risk of infection
- Incomplete emptying
- Instrumentation of the urinary tract or catheters
- Stones
- Glycosuria.

Investigations
- Culture and sensitivity
- Check postvoid residual
- Cystoscopy
- Consider imaging for structural abnormality or evidence of upper tract sequelae, e.g. cortical scarring.

Management
- Adequate fluid intake (often an issue in older people)
- Perineal hygiene:
  - Wiping 'front to back'
  - Postcoital voiding
  - Avoid use of spermicides (toxic effect on normal vaginal flora)
- Topical oestrogen if peri/postmenopausal
- Antibiotic options:
  - Short course
  - Extended prophylaxis
  - Postcoital single dose if clear precipitant
  - Self-start course
- Non-antibiotic treatments: some evidence for D-Mannose (a naturally occurring sugar) and Methenamine (Hiprex®).

❶ Work is currently underway to evaluate options for a vaccine against recurrent UTIs.

Non-bacterial cystitis

Infectious
- Chlamydia
- Mycobacteria
- Fungal—suggests immunocompromise
- Schistosomiasis—long-term infection may cause reduced capacity, obstruction, and bladder cancer.

Drug induced cystitis
Thought to be due to secretion of active metabolites in urine.
    Causative agents include:
- Cyclophosphamide
- Methotrexate
- Allopurinol
- Ketamine—causes fibrosis and severe symptoms (LUTS, pain, haematuria).

Radiation cystitis
- 15–20% patients treated with external beam radiation will experience bladder symptoms
- Onset may be early or late (years after treatment)
- Acute symptoms include haematuria and pain (haemorrhagic cystitis)
- Later symptoms represent ischaemic fibrosis and reduced bladder capacity.

Environmental toxins
    Can cause haemorrhagic cystitis. Implicated in malignancy.
- Aniline dyes
- Toluidine (pesticide)
- Chlordimeform (pesticide).

Inflammatory conditions
- Amyloidosis
- SLE
- Eosinophilic cystitis.

Bladder pain syndrome

ICS definition of bladder pain syndrome
- Suprapubic pain related to bladder filling, accompanied by other symptoms, such as increased daytime and night-time frequency, in the absence of any identifiable pathology or infection.
- 'Interstitial cystitis' was characterized by typical cystoscopic findings of Hunner's ulcers and petechial haemorrhage, but these diagnostic criteria were deemed too strict, leading to underdiagnosis, hence the term 'bladder pain syndrome' was adopted.

Prevalence and aetiology
- Chronic condition of unknown aetiology
- More common in females
- Hard to estimate prevalence due to lack of diagnostic test, estimated at 2.3–6.5%
- Best viewed as a chronic pain condition rather than an inflammatory bladder disorder
- Association with other chronic conditions such as fibromyalgia, vulvodynia, endometriosis, chronic fatigue, and irritable bowel syndrome.

Symptoms
- Pain—bladder, urethra, vagina
- Pain often relieved by voiding
- LUTS—frequency, urgency, constant sensation of needing to void.

Differential diagnosis
Diagnosis of exclusion. Consider:
- Infection
- OAB
- Non-bacterial cystitis
- Endometriosis
- Stones
- Incomplete emptying.

Assessment
- Physical examination for trigger points, bladder distension
- Frequency volume chart—typically small volume
- Urinalysis and culture
- Test for chlamydia and ureaplasma if sterile pyuria
- Cytology if haematuria
- Cystoscopy/cystodistension—to exclude other pathology and may result in temporary relief of symptoms. Typical findings include small capacity bladder, postdistension glomerulation, and haemorrhage. Poor correlation between findings and symptoms
- Biopsy is not needed for diagnosis but may be needed to exclude other pathology.

Management of bladder pain syndrome

Conservative
- Pain management
- Diet (avoid caffeine, alcohol, acidic food)
- Stress management, e.g. exercise, acupuncture
- Support groups
- Physiotherapy.

Pharmacological
- Amitriptyline
- Cimetidine (antihistamine).

Intravesical
- DMSO
- Heparin
- Botulinum toxin A
- Lidocaine
- Chondroitin sulphate
- Hyaluronic acid.

Other
- Pain clinic
- Psychological support
- Neuromodulation (PTNS, SNS)
- Oral cyclosporin A.

Surgical
- Cystodistension (pain relief usually temporary)
- Laser fulguration/resection of Hunner's lesions
- Cystectomy and diversion (last resort).

Not recommended:
- Long-term antibiotics
- Long duration cystodistension
- Intravesical BCG
- Oral glucocorticoids.

Resources
➔ Management of Bladder Pain Syndrome (RCOG Green-top guideline No. 70, 2016).

Urethral conditions

Urethral masses
- Caruncle
- Prolapse
- Malignancy—transitional cell carcinoma, squamous cell carcinoma, sarcoma
- Condylomata
- Polyp
- Fibroid
- Skene's gland cyst or abscess
- Diverticulum.

Caruncle
- Eversion of portion of distal urethra
- Appearance is smooth, fleshy, bright red
- Typically postmenopausal patient
- Presentation: lump, bleeding. May be asymptomatic
- Treatment: topical oestrogen, rarely cautery or excision.

Prolapse
- Circumferential urethral eversion
- Occurs in prepubertal girls and postmenopausal women
- Presentation: bleeding, lump felt
- Treatment: topical oestrogen, surgical excision.

Urethral diverticulum
- Outpouching of urethra into anterior vaginal wall
- Presentation: classic triad of dyspareunia, dysuria, and postvoid dribble. Also, recurrent UTI, rarely stone formation. May be asymptomatic
- Examination may reveal a mass, compression may result in expression of purulent material from urethra
- Cystoscopy and MRI aid diagnosis
- Treatment: surgical excision with interposition fat pad to reduce the risk of fistula.

Urethral stricture
- Rare in women
- Causes: iatrogenic (surgery/instrumentation/radiation), infection, malignancy
- Presentation: LUTS, hesitancy, poor flow, UTI
- Treatment: dilatation, reconstructive surgery.

Urethral syndrome

- Presentation: frequency, urgency, suprapubic discomfort, feeling of incomplete emptying, dysuria, urethral irritation
- Diagnosis of exclusion (caruncle, UTI, STI)
- Conservative measures include avoiding irritants such as shower gel/ bubble bath and spermicides
- Overlap with BPS
- Medical treatment options: topical oestrogen, amitriptyline, local anaesthetic gel, alpha blockers.

Urinary tract injuries

Bladder injury at caesarean section
▶ Frequency 1:100

Risk factors
- Previous CS (risk increases with each subsequent section)
- Emergency delivery
- Second stage section
- Adhesions
- Prematurity.

Mechanism of injury
- Opening peritoneum (33%)
- Creating bladder flap (43%)
- Uterine incision and delivery (23%)
- Delayed (1%)—thermal injury or suture placement
▶ 95% will be at the bladder dome, 5% at the trigone.

Presentation
- Most will be evident at time of surgery
- Missed injuries present with haematuria, pain, ileus, urinary ascites, or fistula.

Intraoperative repair
- If injury is at the dome, it can be repaired by an experienced obstetrician/gynaecologist
- Injuries to the posterior wall or trigone should be repaired by a urologist and integrity of ureters assessed
- Two-layer approach (mucosa + muscularis and serosa) with interrupted or continuous absorbable suture (polyglactin or poliglecaprone)
- Check repair with methylene blue instillation
- Antibiotic cover intraoperatively
- Leave urethral catheter on free drainage for 7–10 days
- Consider cystogram prior to TWOC to ensure integrity of repair.

Bladder injury at laparoscopy
▶ Risk from 0.02% to 8% depending on procedure.

Risk factors
- Endometriosis
- Fibroids
- Cancer
- Adhesions (previous surgery/infection/inflammatory disease/radiation)
- Severe genital organ prolapse
- Obesity
- Pregnant uterus.

Mechanism
- Entry related—suprapubic port insertion
- Dissection related, e.g. bladder reflection
- Disease related, e.g. endometriotic nodule.

Recognition
- Extravasation of urine
- Visualizing the catheter balloon
- Air-filled catheter bag
- If clinically suspected—methylene blue, consider cystoscopy
- Suspect missed injury if postoperative course not straightforward.

Repair
- Will depend on skill set—laparoscopic closure versus laparotomy
- Interrupted polyglactin or poliglecaprone, two-layer technique
- Antibiotic cover intraoperatively
- Catheter on free drainage 7–14 days (depending on size of injury)
- Cystogram prior to TWOC
- If leak still demonstrated at cystogram, leave catheter further 7 days then reassess.

Reducing the risk
- Empty bladder prior to procedure
- Port insertion under vision
- Bladder may be higher than expected in context of previous caesarean section
- Safe use of electrosurgery.

Retroperitoneal injury
For example, bladder perforation with TVT needle.
- Urine will be contained in retropubic space rather than leaking into peritoneal cavity
- Can be managed conservatively.

Ureteric injury
▶ Commonest cause of litigation against gynaecologists.

Incidence
- Overall 0.5–1%
- Abdominal hysterectomy 7:1000
- Vaginal hysterectomy 2:1000
- Caesarean 3:10 000.

Risk factors
- Extensive pelvic surgery
- Endometriosis
- Fibroids
- Previous radiation
- Adhesions
- Excessive bleeding.

Site of ureteric injury
- Pelvic brim—ureter close to infundibulopelvic ligament
- Lateral to cervix—ureter close to uterine artery, uterosacral/cardinal ligament complex
- Ovarian fossae—e.g. endometriosis surgery, postmenopausal oophorectomy.

Mechanism
- Angulation
- Crush
- Ligation
- Thermal
- Laceration
- Transection
- Resection.

Recognition
- 1/3 identified intraoperatively
- On table retrograde ureteropyelogram
- 2/3 not detected and present with postoperative flank pain, ileus, fever, abdominal distension
- Delayed presentation with fistula, e.g. ureterovaginal fistula following hysterectomy.

Repair
Will depend on timing, method, and site of injury.
- Minor crush or thermal injury may need stenting alone
- Anything more will require formal repair, usually requiring open surgery.

Injury above the pelvic brim
- Ureteroureterostomy (end-to-end anastomosis)
- Transureteroureterostomy (end of injured ureter anastomosed to side of contralateral ureter)

Injury below the pelvic brim
- Ureteroneocystostomy (reimplantation)
- If adequate length maintained the ureter is directly reimplanted into the bladder
- If the ureter is shortened, one of the following techniques is used:

Psoas hitch
- The bladder is incised transversely and mobilized to reach the shortened ureter to achieve a tension-free anastomosis
- The bladder is fixed to the psoas muscle
- The bladder incision is repaired in a vertical manner, which allows 'elongation' of the bladder.

Boari flap
- A wide-based flap is developed by an anterior bladder wall incision
- The flap is brought towards the ureter to achieve a tension-free anastomosis
- The bladder incision is closed in a tubular manner, with to up to 12–15cm of additional length.

Principles of ureteric repair
- Tension free
- Ends of ureter 'spatulated'
- Interrupted absorbable suture material
- Stents inserted to maintain patency
- Consideration of abdominal drain (detect anastomotic leak).

Vesicovaginal fistula

Definition
Abnormal communication between bladder and vagina.

Developing countries
▶ Primarily due to obstructed labour:
- Childbearing before full pelvic growth is achieved
- Malnutrition limits pelvic dimensions resulting in cephalopelvic disproportion
- Poor access to healthcare.

These factors result in a very prolonged second stage, the fetal head causes pressure necrosis of pelvic structures.

Developed countries
▶ Primarily iatrogenic
- 90% due surgical injury (mostly gynaecological procedures, 75% as a result of hysterectomy)
- Radiotherapy
- Foreign body, e.g. neglected pessary
- Rarely infective cause (TB, syphilis).

Risk factors for iatrogenic fistula
- Previous surgery
- PID
- Ischaemia
- Diabetes
- Cancer
- Endometriosis.

Presentation
- Obstetric: develop in first few days
- Surgical: typically 7–30 days postoperative
- Radiotherapy: late (years after treatment)
- Symptoms of continuous urinary incontinence or watery vaginal discharge postsurgery should raise suspicion of VVF.

Assessment
- Large fistulae may be visualized easily
- EUA with cystoscopy
- Imaging—IVU/cystogram
- Dye tests—indigo carmine/methylene blue.

Management
- Catheter on continuous drainage may be sufficient to heal a small VVF if detected early
- Most will require formal repair.

Surgical repair
- Should be undertaken by surgeon with appropriate expertise in centres with significant caseload
- Approach may be abdominal, vaginal, or combined
- Some evidence that interposition grafts reduce risk of recurrence.

Principles of repair
- Accurate diagnosis
- Adequate exposure
- Careful haemostasis
- Mobilization of tissue
- Tension free
- Watertight bladder closure
- Maintain adequate blood supply
- Postoperative catheter to allow healing.

Urinary catheters

Three main types:
- Urethral
- Suprapubic
- Intermittent.

Basics
- Made from latex or silicone
- Catheters for long-term use are coated with hydrophilic polymers which reduced friction and encrustation
- Length: 26cm for females, 42cm for males
- Size: circumference in mm (described as Charrière (Ch) or French (F))
- Channels: 2-way (drainage and balloon) or 3-way (drainage, balloon, and irrigation)
- Balloon: fill with sterile water (sodium chloride may crystallize in the channel and cause deflation failure)
- Flip-flow valve: mimic physiological filling and emptying of bladder.

Suprapubic catheters
- Usually inserted via percutaneous approach with distended bladder and cystoscopic guidance
▶ If previous extensive abdominal/pelvic surgery or if unable to distend bladder an open approach should be used due to the risk of visceral injury.

Advantages of SPC over urethral catheters:
- More comfortable
- Less bypassing
- Easier to be sexually active/less inhibiting.

Disadvantages of SPC compared to urethral catheters:
- Skill required for insertion
- Increased risk of insertion (mortality reported as up to 2%)
- Granulation tissue forms at cystotomy site
- Less time to insert new catheter if falls out (tract starts to close).

Clean intermittent self-catheterization
- Allows freedom from collection systems and ability to empty bladder when socially appropriate/convenient
- Mimic natural filling/voiding pattern
- Low complication rate
- Avoids the complications associated with long-term indwelling catheter use (infection, pain, encrustation, trauma).

Troubleshooting
See Table 5.1.

Table 5.1 Troubleshooting indwelling catheter problems

Problem	Description	Solution
Bypassing	Urine leaking from urethra or cystotomy	• Use correct size catheter • Suppress DO with anticholinergic or Botox
Blockage	Encrustation	• Replace catheter more regularly • Increase fluid intake • Lemon drinks increase citrate in urine
Pain	Eyelet may be occluded by urothelium due to hydrostatic suction	• Raise drainage bag above level of bladder for 15 seconds
Urine not draining	Kinking, incorrect drainage position	• Keep drainage bag below level of bladder
Balloon diffusion	Balloon slowly deflates	• Inflate 100% silicon catheter balloon with 5% aqueous glycerine in 10ml sterile water

Urinary diversion

Indications
- Cystectomy (cancer, intractable pain)
- Neurogenic bladder
- Radiation damage
- Intractable incontinence.

Techniques

Non-continent
- Ileal conduit—ureters drain into small ileal pouch. Pouch forms cutaneous urostomy.

Continent
- Urostomy which can be intermittently catheterized
- Formation of neo-bladder (orthotopic diversion)
- Ureterosigmoidostomy.
- ❶ All may cause issues with metabolic disturbance.

Colorectal

Investigations *112*
Constipation *114*
Obstructed defaecation syndrome (ODS) *116*
Rectal prolapse *118*
Intussusception *120*
Faecal incontinence *122*
Relevant procedures *124*
Rectovaginal fistula (RVF) *126*

Investigations

Endoanal ultrasonography
- See Fig. 6.1
- High sensitivity and specificity
- Used to visualize anal canal musculature
- Assess for sphincter defects.

Evacuating proctogram (defaecography)
- Dynamic examination
- Barium paste is inserted via rectal catheter then video fluoroscopy recording of defaecation
- Use to diagnose:
  - Intussusception
  - Rectocele
  - Rectal prolapse.

Anorectal manometry (physiology)
- Evaluates motor and sensory function of defaecatory unit
- Resting pressure correlates with IAS function
- Squeeze pressure correlates with EAS function.

Transit study
- Assesses the length of food transit through gut
- Patient swallows radio-opaque capsules over a period of time followed by an abdominal X-ray
- Looks for slow transit constipation.

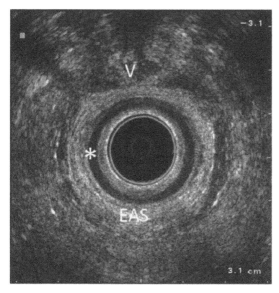

Fig. 6.1 Endoanal ultrasound of mid anal canal: EAS, internal anal sphincter (*), and vagina (V).

Reprinted from Lindsey I et al (2010) *Pelvic floor disorders for the colorectal surgeon* Oxford: Oxford University Press, with permission from Oxford University Press

Constipation

- Patients and medical professionals vary in their use of the word constipation—some mean infrequent passage of stool, others mean passage of very hard stool.
- Normal bowel habit varies from 3 times a day to 3 times a week.

Medical definition

Fewer than 3 bowel motions a week, plus 2 of the following:
- Straining
- Hard stool
- Need to digitate/support perineum
- Repeated visits to achieve emptying
- Feeling of incomplete emptying.

Causes—lifestyle
- Dietary
- Insufficient fluid intake
- Insufficient activity
- Stress
- Ignoring the urge to go—over time results in loss of sensitivity to gastro-colic reflex
- Shift work
- Lack of privacy and/or 'safe toilet environment'
- Pregnancy/recent childbirth.

Causes—medications
Many medications cause constipation as a side effect. Some common culprits include:
- Opiates
- Aluminium-containing antacids
- Iron
- Antimuscarinics
- Antihistamines
- Tricyclic antidepressants
- Calcium supplements
- Diuretics
- Antidiarrhoeal medication.

Causes—medical conditions
- Irritable bowel syndrome
- Pain around the anus, e.g. fissures, postsurgery
- Hypothyroidism
- Hypercalcaemia
- Spinal injury
- Bowel tumours
- Neurological conditions, e.g. multiple sclerosis, Parkinson's disease
- Depression
- Slow transit
- Obstructive defaecation.

Assessment
- Thorough history
- Examination including digital rectal examination
- Proctogram to assess for evacuatory disorder if symptoms suggestive
- Transit study.

🚫 If red flags present, patient needs colonoscopy or CT colonoscopy to exclude malignancy.

Management
Will depend on underlying cause.
  Symptomatic treatments include:
- Dietary—including enough of the right type of fibre
- Fluid—minimum of 1.5L non-caffeinated fluid per day
- Increase physical activity
- Routine—allowing time and privacy for bowel movements
- Position—using a footstool, leaning forward
- Laxatives—➲ see next section.
- Rectal irrigation systems
- Surgery for obstructive causes
- Subtotal colectomy is now rarely performed as results are mixed.

Laxatives
Natural fibres
Bulk forming
- Golden linseed
- Psyllium or ispaghula husk (Fybogel, Regulan)
- Require good fluid intake as the fibre absorbs water

Osmotic
Increase water content of stool.
- Sorbitol—contained in diet products, prunes, dried fruit
- Lactulose—can cause excess gas production
- Macrogols (Movicol, Laxido)—cause less bloating than lactulose

Stimulant
Increase intestinal motility
- Senna, bisacodyl, sodium picosulfate
- Co-danthramer—only for use in terminally ill patients as potentially carcinogenic
- May cause cramping
- Should be avoided if obstruction suspected.

Faecal softeners
Decrease surface tension and increase fluid penetration into faecal mass
- Docusate sodium
- Arachis oil enemas.

Others
- Prucalopride (Resolor)—acts directly on the nervous system of the gastrointestinal tract
- Lubiprostone—chloride channel activator
- Glycerine suppositories—cause rectal stimulation, faecal softener, plus lubricating properties.

Obstructed defaecation syndrome (ODS)

Causes of ODS
- Intussusception
- Rectal prolapse
- Rectocele or enterocoele
- Anismus.

History
- Difficulty passing motions, straining
- Repeated, unsuccessful attempts to pass stool
- Sensation of blockage/incomplete emptying
- Digitating rectally or vaginally.

▶ Symptoms tend to worsen with age as connective tissue weakens.

Examination
- Perineum—scars, deficiency
- Vaginal—prolapse
- Rectal—prolapse, squeeze, tone.

Investigations
- Flexible sigmoidoscopy/colonoscopy
- Endoanal ultrasound—may show thickened IAS
- Anorectal physiology
- Defaecating proctogram
- Transit studies.

Management
- Dietary changes
- Bulking agents
- Pelvic floor retraining
- Biofeedback
- Irrigation
- Repair of anatomical defect—repair rectocele, rectopexy, transanal repair.

Rectal prolapse

- Rectum loses proper attachment and telescopes downwards
- Can be full thickness (rectal wall) or mucosal
- Worse with increased intra-abdominal pressure.

Risk factors for rectal prolapse
- Vaginal births
- Chronic constipation
- Hysterectomy
- Weak connective tissue/hypermobility

Symptoms
- ODS
- Lump protruding
- Pain
- Incontinence (stretching of sphincter muscles plus damage to pudendal nerves).

Management
- Dietary measures
- Pelvic floor retraining
- Laparoscopic ventral rectopexy
- Stapled transanal resection of rectum (STARR)
- Sutured transanal mucosectomy and plication (STAMP)
- Anterior Delorme's procedure.

Intussusception

- Also called internal rectal prolapse
- Rectum telescopes down within the rectum (low grade) or anal canal (high grade).

▶ 90% are female, strongly related to childbirth.

Symptoms
- ODS
- Pain
- Incontinence.

Investigation
- Defaecating proctogram
- Physiology.

Management
- Dietary measures
- Pelvic floor retraining
- Laparoscopic ventral rectopexy.

Grading
See Table 6.1.

Table 6.1 Oxford grading system for rectal prolapse

Rectal intussusception	Grade I	Descends no lower than the proximal limit of the rectocele
	Grade II	Descends into the level of the rectocele, but not to the anal canal
Rectoanal intussusception	Grade III	Descends to the top of the anal canal
	Grade IV	Descends into the anal canal
External rectal prolapse	Grade V	Protrudes from the anus

Faecal incontinence

- Loss of control over passage of stool or flatus
- Affects 10–15% of adults
- May be urgent, passive, or postdefaecatory.

❶ Adverse consequences are physical, psychological, social, and economic.

Causes of faecal incontinence

Sphincter/pelvic floor damage
- Obstetric
- Iatrogenic (e.g. following anorectal surgery)
- Trauma
- Congenital

Anorectal pathology
- Prolapse
- Fistula

Neurological
- Spina bifida
- Pudendal neuropathy
- CNS—tumour, trauma, stroke
- Dementia

Gastrointestinal
- Inflammatory bowel disease
- IBS
- Radiotherapy
- Laxative abuse
- Overflow (faecal impaction)
- Drug related
- Dietary
- Tumour.

History
- Consistency of stool
- Differentiate urge from passive from postdefaecatory (may overlap)
- Symptoms questionnaires, e.g. St Mark's Incontinence Score.

Examination
- Pelvic floor assessment
- Gaping of anus on Valsalva
- Rectal—tone, stool, tumour.

Investigations
- Sigmoidoscopy/proctoscopy
- Endoanal ultrasound
- Anorectal physiology.

Management of faecal incontinence

Conservative

- Dietary manipulation
- Fluid: reduce caffeine and fizzy drinks
- Physiotherapy and bowel retraining
- Biofeedback
- Loperamide
- Anal plugs
- Pads
- Rectal irrigation.

Surgical

Sphincteroplasty

- For EAS defect
- Uses anterior overlapping technique
- Achieves 60–80% continence.

Sacral nerve stimulation

- Low level stimulation to sacral nerves, stimulating the pelvic floor and EAS
- Test wire first, permanent implant if effective.

Gracioplasty

- Gracilis muscle transposed and electrically stimulated, converting fibres from skeletal to smooth muscle.

Artificial anal sphincter

- High morbidity and explant rates.

Diversion

- End colostomy.

Relevant procedures

Anterior Delorme's procedure
- *Use*: rectal prolapse, rectocele
- *Technique*: Transanal approach to rectovaginal septum. Mucosa dissected from muscle, muscle plicated, mucosa trimmed and sutured.

Stapled transanal resection of rectum (STARR)
- *Use*: ODS caused by intussusception
- *Technique*: Transanal approach. Staple device removes loose rectal wall.

Sutured transanal mucosectomy and plication (STAMP)
- *Use*: simultaneously repair rectocele and mucosal prolapse
- *Technique*: Transanal approach. Similar to anterior Delorme's but circumferential correction.

Laparoscopic ventral rectopexy
- *Use*: external rectal prolapse and intussusception causing ODS or incontinence
- *Technique*: polypropylene mesh sutured to anterior rectum and fixed to sacral promontory.

Rectovaginal fistula (RVF)

An abnormal, epithelial lined connection between vagina and rectum.

Causes
- Obstetric lacerations—failure to identify/repair or breakdown
- Obstructed labour causing pressure necrosis
- Complication of surgery—STARR, stapled haemorrhoidectomy, rectocele repair
- Trauma
- Diverticulitis
- Inflammatory bowel disease
- Malignancy
- Radiotherapy.

Symptoms
- Passage of stool/flatus PV
- Offensive PV discharge
- Recurrent vaginitis.

Assessment
- Careful examination—may need EUA
- MRI
- Barium enema

▶Assessment of continence is required—may be difficult to assess on symptoms alone.

Management of RVF
- Small defects may heal spontaneously
- Larger defects likely to need surgical closure
- Technique will depend on aetiology but may be transanal, transvaginal, or transabdominal
- Diversion may be required to allow healing.

Neurology

Overview *128*
Brain lesions *130*
Spinal cord lesions *132*
Sacral cord injuries *134*
Peripheral neuropathy *136*

Overview

▶ Impact on bladder function and upper renal tract depends on the site of the lesion.

• Interruption of inhibitory pathways from the cerebral cortex to the pontine micturition centre is likely to result in uninhibited detrusor contractions
e.g. stroke, tumours, Parkinson's disease.

• Interruption of neural pathways from the pontine to the sacral centres leads to uninhibited detrusor contractions with or without failure of relaxation of the urethral sphincter (detrusor sphincter dyssynergia)
e.g. multiple sclerosis, cord injury.

• Interruption of sacral reflex arc leads to acontractility of the detrusor muscle and atony with voiding difficulty
e.g. diabetic neuropathy, lumbar disc prolapse.

❶ The combination of a high-pressure bladder with failure of relaxation of the urethral sphincter will result in vesicoureteric reflux, dilatation of the upper tracts, and ultimately renal damage unless managed carefully.

Resources

➔ NICE Clinical guideline [CG148]. Urinary incontinence in neurological disease: assessment and management. August 2012.

Brain lesions

▶ Lesions above the pons affect higher conscious control of voiding but primitive voiding reflexes remain intact. Typically, symptoms are those of frequency, urgency, urge incontinence, and nocturia and they should respond to standard management of OAB.

Stroke

• Initial acute phase of cerebral shock results in detrusor areflexia and urinary retention
• Subsequent detrusor hyperreflexia results in frequency, urgency, and urge incontinence.

Frontal lobe lesions

• e.g. Dementia, tumour
• Socially inappropriate micturition or defaecation
• Voluntary act rather than true incontinence
• Lack of awareness of 'acceptable' voiding.

Parkinson's disease

• Dopamine deficiency and increased cholinergic activity in corpus stratum
• Detrusor hyperreflexia is combined with bradykinesia of the urethral sphincter
• Variable response to L-dopa
• Often intractable constipation due to autonomic dysfunction.

Multiple systems atrophy

• Parkinson's like symptoms, cerebellar ataxia, and autonomic dysfunction
• Degeneration of the nucleus of Onuf results in denervation of the external striated sphincter
• Open bladder neck due to sympathetic nerve atrophy
• Initial symptoms of detrusor hyperreflexia, but develop atonic bladder over years of disease progression.

Spinal cord lesions

▶ Symptoms will depend on site and mechanism of injury.

Spinal cord trauma

Initial phase of spinal shock results in detrusor areflexia and urinary retention (usually lasts 6–12 weeks). Subsequently detrusor hyperreflexia develops with detrusor sphincter dyssynergia.

Lesions above T6
- Detrusor hyperreflexia, striated, and smooth sphincter dyssynergia
- Autonomic dysreflexia—exaggerated sympathetic response to stimuli below the level of the cord injury, e.g. distended bladder or catheterization.

Lesions below T6
- As for higher lesions but without autonomic dysreflexia.

Management
- Indwelling catheter for initial spinal shock
- Subsequently may prefer intermittent catheterization combined with treatment to suppress detrusor contractions, e.g. anticholinergics, botulinum toxin.

Multiple sclerosis

Focal demyelinating lesions of the central nervous system, usually involving posterior and lateral columns of the spinal cord. Most women with MS will experience some degree of lower urinary tract dysfunction. In a minority, urinary symptoms may be the initial presenting feature.
- Commonest urodynamic finding is detrusor hyperreflexia
- May be associated with detrusor sphincter dyssynergia
- 25% display detrusor areflexia
- UTIs are common if emptying is impaired which may aggravate other MS symptoms.

Management
- Will depend on symptoms and urodynamic findings
- Anticholinergics and botulinum toxin are useful for detrusor hyperreflexia
- Clean intermittent catheterization is used for voiding dysfunction.

Sacral cord injuries

Two main impacts:
- Loss of bladder sensation
- Detrusor areflexia

This results in retention and overflow incontinence.

Causes

- Sacral cord tumour
- Herniated disc
- Pelvic crush injury.

Peripheral neuropathy

Diabetes
- Bladder dysfunction typically appears 10y after diagnosis
- Autonomic and peripheral neuropathy
- Loss of sensation of filling is followed by reduced contractility
- Symptoms of reduced filling sensation, poor emptying, recurrent UTI
- Eventual detrusor areflexia.

Herpes zoster
- Neuropathy with painful vesicles over the distribution of the nerve
- Sacral nerve involvement leads to impaired detrusor function
- Early stages—urgency, frequency, urge incontinence
- Late stages—decreased bladder sensation, incomplete emptying, retention
- Self-limiting—symptoms resolve with clearance of the infection.

Pelvic surgery
Extensive pelvic surgery may result in bladder dysfunction in the form of detrusor areflexia, e.g. radical hysterectomy, abdominoperineal resection, exenteration. 80% will recover spontaneously but this takes months.

Pregnancy and childbirth

Physiological changes of pregnancy *138*
Perineal trauma *140*
Obstetric anal sphincter injury *142*
Postpartum urinary retention *144*

Physiological changes of pregnancy

Renal tract
- Kidney volume increase by up to 30%
- ↑ renal plasma flow
- ↑ GFR
- Dilatation of renal pelvis and ureter in 80% women, right > left (progesterone effect plus mechanical compression at pelvic brim); resolves by 6–8 weeks postdelivery.

Bladder
- The mucosa will be oedematous and hyperaemic
- Progesterone causes bladder relaxation
- The bladder is displaced superiorly and anteriorly by the uterus which may ↓ capacity
- Bladder flaccidity results in intermittent ureteric reflux.

Pelvic floor
- Progesterone relaxes muscles
- Pressure from gravid uterus
- Constipation can put additional pressure on pelvic floor.

Bladder symptoms in pregnancy
- ↑ frequency and nocturia are common (>80%) and need no treatment
- Urinary stasis results in increased rates of asymptomatic bacteriuria, UTI, and pyelonephritis.

❶ Untreated UTI is associated with maternal and fetal morbidity (preterm birth, low birthweight).

Perineal trauma

▶It is estimated that over 85% of women delivering vaginally will sustain some form of perineal tear.

Classification of perineal trauma

First-degree tear
Injury to the perineal skin or vaginal mucosa.

Second-degree tear
Injury to perineum involving perineal muscles but not involving the anal sphincter.

Third-degree tear
Injury to the perineum involving the anal sphincter complex.
• 3a: <50% external anal sphincter (EAS) torn
• 3b: >50% EAS torn
• 3c: Both EAS and internal anal sphincter (IAS) torn

Fourth-degree tear
Injury to perineum involving the anal sphincter complex (EAS and IAS) and anorectal mucosa.

Rectal buttonhole tear
Tear of the rectal mucosa with intact sphincter complex.

Obstetric anal sphincter injury (OASI)
Third- and fourth-degree tears.

Episiotomy

This may be mediolateral (beginning from the posterior fourchette and directed at an angle of 45° to the midline, see Fig. 8.1) or midline (following the natural line of the perineal muscles). Mediolateral incisions result in more blood loss, pain, and dyspareunia, but midline incisions have a higher risk of injuring the anal sphincter.

▶For every 6° the episiotomy is made away from the midline, there is a 50% reduction in OASI.

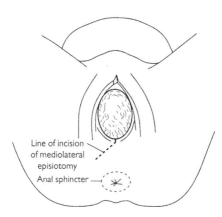

Fig. 8.1 Cutting an episiotomy.

Reprinted from Collins S et al (2013) *Oxford Handbook of Obstetrics and Gynaecology* 3rd edition, Oxford University Press, adapted from the original in Wyatt JP et al (2006) *Oxford Handbook of Emergency Medicine* Oxford: Oxford University Press, with permission from Oxford University Press

Obstetric anal sphincter injury

Normal anal sphincter
Complex of EAS and IAS.

EAS
- Striated muscle innervated by pudendal nerve
- Under voluntary control
- Accounts for 25–30% resting tone and 70% squeeze pressure.

IAS
- Continuation of circular smooth muscle of colon, under autonomic control
- Accounts for 70% resting tone

▶ Damage to the IAS is more predictive of anal incontinence than damage to the EAS.

Risk factors for OASI
- First vaginal birth
- Persistent OP position
- Birthweight >4000g
- Induction of labour
- 2nd stage >1h
- Shoulder dystocia
- Midline episiotomy
- Forceps delivery
- Epidural analgesia.

Identification of injury
- Systematic examination by experienced practitioner
- Inspect:
  - Absent puckering around anus
  - EAS looks like 'red meat'
  - IAS looks like pale circular fibres
- Feel:
  - Anal squeeze
  - 'Pill rolling' technique to assess sphincter.

Repair of injury—general principles
- Repair should take place in theatre
- Repair should be by an appropriately trained practitioner or by a trainee under supervision
- A rectal examination should be performed after the repair to ensure no sutures have passed through the anorectal mucosa.

Repair of injury—technique
- Anorectal mucosa—3-0 polyglactin either interrupted or continuous.
- IAS—should be repaired separate to the EAS as this improves future anal continence. 2-0 polyglactin or 3-0 PDS may be used. An end-to-end technique is preferred.

- EAS—there is no difference in outcome between overlapping and end-to-end techniques. For partial thickness tears overlapping will not be possible and so an end-to-end approach should be used. 2-0 polyglactin or 3-0 PDS may be used with equivalent outcomes.

Postoperative management
- Broad-spectrum antibiotic reduces the risk of infection
- Laxatives reduce the risk of wound dehiscence. Bulking agents should not be given with laxatives
- Physiotherapy may be beneficial
- Patients should be reviewed at 6–12 weeks postdelivery. If there is ongoing pain or incontinence, referral to a specialized gynaecologist or colorectal surgeon is recommended.

Prognosis
Approx. 60–80% of women are asymptomatic at 12 months after EAS repair.

Future delivery
- There are no RCTs or systematic reviews to guide mode of delivery following OASI.
- The risk of a further OASI is 5–7%, and 17% experience worsening faecal symptoms following a second vaginal birth.
- Prophylactic episiotomy does not prevent OASI and is not recommended.
- If the woman is symptomatic or shows abnormally low anorectal manometric pressures and/or endoanal ultrasonographic defects, an elective caesarean section may be considered.

Resources
➲ Third- and Fourth-degree Perineal Tears, Management (RCOG Green-top Guideline No. 29, 2015).

Postpartum urinary retention

▶Affects 10–15% of patients.

Two types

- *Overt*—the inability to void spontaneously within 6h of vaginal birth or removal of indwelling catheter
- *Covert*—postvoid residual volumes of >150ml. May be asymptomatic.

Risk factors

- Prior history of voiding difficulties
- Primiparity
- First vaginal birth
- Epidural, spinal, or pudendal block in labour
- Difficult instrumental birth
- Shoulder dystocia
- Prolonged second stage
- Birth weight of >3.8kg
- Excessive perineal trauma or oedema.

Symptoms/signs

- Cannot void/failed TWOC
- Straining to void
- Poor flow/dribbling
- Incontinence
- Reduced sensation
- Deviated uterus
- Increased blood loss
- May or may not be painful.

Mechanism

Physiological

- High progesterone levels in pregnancy reduce detrusor tone
- Therefore, the bladder is already hypotonic and vulnerable to further insult
- Postpartum diuresis is common.

Mechanical

- Oedema of vulva/urethra
- Overdistension of bladder further reduces contractility.

Neurological

- Pressure/stretching of pelvic and pudendal nerves.

Consequences

- UTI
- Incontinence (overflow)
- Short- and long-term bladder dysfunction
- Ureteric reflux
- Hydronephrosis
- Renal impairment.

❶ A single episode of bladder overdistension can permanently affect the ability of the detrusor to contract, resulting in long-term voiding dysfunction. The higher the volume, the worse the prognosis.

Prevention
- Intrapartum: monitor fluid balance, aim for 4-hourly voids, offer catheter if unable to spontaneously void
- Postpartum: measure and document first void, aim for void within 4h of delivery/removal of catheter.

Management
- Conservative measures to promote voiding
  - Analgesia
  - Privacy
  - Void in the shower/bath
  - Treat constipation
  - Timed voiding if reduced sensation
  - Physiotherapy input
- Catheters
  - Follow local protocols
  - If fail initial TWOC, consider either indwelling catheter with flip-flow valve or intermittent self-catheterization.

Age and the pelvic floor

Incontinence in children *148*
Urinary tract infection in children *150*
The menopause *152*
Incontinence in the elderly *154*

Incontinence in children

- >90% of children will be dry in the day by the age of 5.
- Nocturnal enuresis affects 10% of 7 year olds, 3% of 12 year olds, and 1% of 18 year olds.

Causes of daytime incontinence

- Constipation (implicated in >70%)
- UTI
- Excessive consumption of caffeine/fizzy drinks/blackcurrant drinks
- Bladder overactivity
- Anxiety or emotional upset
- Incomplete emptying (commonly related to position on toilet—feet not touching the floor)
- Delaying voiding—may be due to concentrating on playing/forgetting to go or due to toilet phobias
- Diabetes
- Anatomical anomalies—ectopic ureter, labial adhesions (urine pools in vagina then dribbles)
- Neurological.

Treatment

- Depends on cause, but will usually involve lifestyle modifications such as managing constipation, fluid intake, and timed toileting
- Anticholinergic treatment may be considered if behavioural modification is unsuccessful.

Nocturnal enuresis (bedwetting)

A number of factors may contribute:

- Ability to concentrate urine overnight may be immature
- Not waking with bladder sensation
- Overactive bladder contractions
- Change in home circumstances, anxiety, or emotional upset can be a trigger.

Treatment

- Reward systems
- Alarms
- Desmopressin if inability to concentrate is suspected
- If there are coexisting daytime symptoms suggesting overactivity, then anticholinergics may be used.

Giggle incontinence

- Common in girls
- Can be large volume
- Mechanism unclear, some evidence to suggest laughter provokes a detrusor contraction
- Usually no treatment needed other than behavioural modification.

Urinary tract infection in children

Presentation
- Urinary symptoms may be present such as frequency, dysuria, offensive urine, or incontinence in a previously dry child.

❶ Symptoms may be non-specific, e.g. vomiting, pyrexia, lethargy, poor feeding, abdominal pain.

Atypical UTI
- Child may be seriously ill
- Poor urine flow
- Associated abdominal mass
- Raised creatinine
- No response to treatment in 48h
- Non-*E. Coli* organisms.

Recurrent UTI
- Two or more episodes of UTI with acute pyelonephritis/upper urinary tract infection, or
- One episode of UTI with acute pyelonephritis/upper urinary tract infection plus one or more episode of UTI with cystitis/lower urinary tract infection, or
- Three or more episodes of UTI with cystitis/lower urinary tract infection.

Investigation
- Investigate all atypical and recurrent UTIs
- Clean catch urine sample
- USS renal tract and bladder (assess anatomy, renal cortical thickness)
- Isotope renography (assess for renal parenchymal defect)
- May consider micturating cystourethrogram if reflux suspected.

Resources
➲ NICE Clinical guideline [CG54]. Urinary tract infection in under 16s: diagnosis and management. Published 2007, updated 2018.

The menopause

Impact on the urogenital tract
- Hormonal changes have a significant impact on oestrogen-sensitive tissue
- Oestrogen receptors are found in the squamous epithelium of the urethra, vagina, trigone, and levator ani muscle
- Reduced oestrogen levels lead to a reduction in the number of epithelial cells being produced, causing thinning of tissues
- Fibroblasts are also oestrogen sensitive, and in its absence produce less collagen, leading to reduced tissue elasticity
- These atrophic changes lead to multiple symptoms.

Common lower urinary tract symptoms
- Frequency
- Nocturia
- Urgency
- Incontinence
- Recurrent UTI
- Urethritis.

Common vulvovaginal symptoms
- Dryness
- Pruritis
- Burning
- Discharge
- Dyspareunia
- Prolapse
The vulva and vagina will typically look pale with loss of rugae.

Treatment
- Topical oestrogen treatment (pessaries or cream) is used in preference to systemic treatment
- Topical oestrogen should be used nightly for 2–4 weeks to address symptoms, then used 2–3 times weekly as maintenance therapy

▶ Patients should be reassured that topical oestrogen does not have the same risk profile as systemic HRT and can be used indefinitely.

Effect of oestrogen on the lower urinary tract
- ↑ urethral closure pressure
- Stimulates periurethral collagen production
- Improved neural control of the bladder
- ↑ sensory threshold of the bladder
- ↓ UTI.

Recurrent UTI in postmenopausal women

Causes:
- Impaired bladder emptying
- Altered vaginal flora (↑ pH)
- Loss of collagen leading to impaired barrier function.
▶ Simple UTIs should respond well to topical oestrogen therapy.

❶ Red flag symptoms require further investigation, including:
- Haematuria
- Persistent bladder pain.

Incontinence in the elderly

Scope of the problem
- Affects more than 1/5 of over 85s (but is under-reported)
- Multifactorial
- Detrusor function reduces with age
- Older people are more likely to delay seeking help (embarrassment, belief that leakage is inevitable and not soluble)
- Urinary incontinence is secondary only to dementia as a reason for admission to long-term care
- Often poorly managed in primary and secondary care.

▶ Incontinence in the elderly is associated with significant morbidity
- Damage to skin integrity
- Recurrent UTI
- Increased risk of falls
- Psychological distress and isolation.

Types of incontinence
- Stress incontinence
- Urge incontinence
- Overflow incontinence
- Functional incontinence (reduced mobility or cognition)
- Mixed
- Transient (due to constipation, UTI, temporary reduction in mobility).

Diagnosis
Usually confirmed by history, examination, and simple investigations.
- Urine dipstick and MSU for culture
- Bladder diary
- Postvoid residual
- Urodynamic assessment may be indicated if initial treatment fails
- Low threshold for cystoscopy.

Treatment considerations
- Polypharmacy
- Comorbidities
- Mobility—need for continence aids such as pads or commodes, risk of falls

▶ May be best treated in conjunction with a care of the elderly physician.

Laparoscopic urogynaecology

Overview *156*
Patient selection *158*
Laparoscopic entry *160*
Laparoscopic procedures *162*
Training in laparoscopic urogynaecology *164*

Overview

▶ Laparoscopic surgery is well-established in the management of benign gynaecological conditions, and is increasing in use in urogynaecology.

Advantages of laparoscopic surgery—patient

- Smaller incisions—reduced wound complications, better cosmesis
- Less analgesic requirement
- Shorter hospital stay
- Less adhesion formation
- Reduced blood loss.

Advantages of laparoscopic surgery—surgeon

- Magnified view
- Easier access to deep pelvis.

Disadvantages of laparoscopic surgery

- Steep learning curve as compared to open surgery
- Initial operating times will be longer until competence is attained
- In the event of haemorrhage, the laparoscopic view is quickly lost and a low threshold is needed to open in these rare cases.

Patient selection

As with any surgery, patient selection is key. There are some patients where special consideration is needed:

Adhesions

- Patients who have had previous abdominal surgery may have intraperitoneal adhesions, particularly in the case of midline open surgery, e.g. bowel resection.
- Other patients who may have adhesions include those with inflammatory bowel disease or peritonitis.
- The umbilicus is a frequent site of bowel adhesions (50% if previous midline, 23% if lower transverse incision).
- Palmer's point (3cm below the left costal margin in the midclavicular line) should be used for the primary trocar if there is suspicion of adhesions at the umbilicus.

Obesity

- Obese women are at higher risk of complications from open surgery (thrombosis, wound infection, etc.), and so minimal access surgery may be of particular benefit.
- Once pneumoperitoneum is established surgery is often straightforward.
- Pneumoperitoneum and head-down positioning may make ventilation more difficult.

Low BMI

- The aorta may lie less than 2.5cm from the skin in very thin women and particular care with entry is required.
▶ Young nulliparous women with high muscle tone are at the highest risk from entry-related vascular injuries.

Age

- There is a perception that laparoscopic surgery should be the preserve of younger patients, but recent data suggests it is usually tolerated well in the elderly provided they are fit for general anaesthesia.

Anaesthetic considerations

- Pneumoperitoneum and head-down positions put increased pressure on the cardiovascular system.
- High airway pressures and carbon dioxide levels may be of particular concern.
- Challenging patients include the obese, those with airway disease, or severe ischaemic heart disease.

Laparoscopic entry

🛈 Serious complications occur approximately 1:1000 laparoscopies, with most occurring as a result of trocar insertion.

▶ A laparoscopic surgeon should be familiar with different techniques for entry.

Veress needle

- Most commonly used technique in gynaecological laparoscopy
- Closed technique
- The abdomen is insufflated with carbon dioxide prior to trocar insertion
- Insertion may be at the umbilicus or Palmer's point
- Palmer's point entry is recommended if there is suspicion of midline adhesions and in morbid obesity. It should also be considered in very thin patients to reduce the risk of vascular injury.

Hasson entry

- More frequently used by general surgeons
- Open technique
- Avoids the use of sharp instruments after the initial incision and allows insertion of a blunt trocar under direct vision.

▶ A meta-analysis of both techniques does not suggest any safety advantage to either method.

Resources

➔ Preventing entry-related gynaecological laparoscopic injuries (RCOG Green-top Guidance No. 49, 2008).

Laparoscopic procedures

Laparoscopic procedures for prolapse

- Laparoscopic hysteropexy
- Laparoscopic sacrocolpopexy
- Laparoscopic paravaginal repair.
- ➲ See Chapter 4, Pelvic organ prolapse, for operative details.

Laparoscopic procedures for SUI

- Laparoscopic colposuspension
- ➲ See Chapter 3, Lower urinary tract conditions, for operative details.

Laparoscopic excision of mesh

- Removal of mid-urethral slings
- Removal of abdominally inserted mesh for prolapse.

Laparoscopic management of complications

- Washout of pelvic haematoma, e.g. vaginal vault haematoma following hysterectomy.

Training in laparoscopic urogynaecology

- Laparoscopic urogynaecology is becoming more widespread and the training curricula is changing to reflect this.
- It is now a mandatory part of subspecialty training.
- A new ATSM in 'Laparoscopic urogynaecology' is available for those undertaking or who have completed the ATSM in 'Urogynaecology and vaginal surgery'.

Tips for training

- Skills from benign gynaecology are readily transferrable.
- Use of laparoscopic box trainers and virtual reality simulators mean that many skills can be acquired outside of the operating theatre.
- 'Buddy' operating is a valuable resource.

Resources

⌨ https://www.rcog.org.uk/en/careers-training/specialty-training-curriculum/

Miscellaneous

What is a urogynaecologist? *166*
Training in urogynaecology *168*
The multidisciplinary team (MDT) *170*
Mesh in urogynaecology *172*

What is a urogynaecologist?

Definition
See Box 11.1.

> **Box 11.1 Definition of a urogynaecologist**
>
> The British Society of Urogynaecology defines a urogynaecologist as a specialist who meets the following criteria:
> - Dedicated urogynaecology clinic or equivalent per week including secondary and tertiary referrals, as part of a multidisciplinary service.
> - Evidence of training in a unit which provides the full range of investigations and treatments required for training.
> - Urodynamics experience, e.g. special skills training.
> - Regular urodynamic sessions (minimum of one per month) either personally or in a supervisory capacity.
> - Provide three clinical sessions in urogynaecology per week.
> - One major urogynaecology procedure associated with pelvic floor dysfunction, i.e. incontinence and prolapse per working week per year.
> - Audit, e.g. BSUG surgical audit.
> - Proportion of continuing medical education in urogynaecology.
>
> Reprinted with kind permission from The British Society of Urogynaecology, available at https://bsug.org.uk/pages/about/definition-of-urogynaecologist/84

Training in urogynaecology

Specialty training programme

All UK specialty trainees in Obstetrics and Gynaecology are required to complete a core curriculum module (2013 curriculum, updated 2016) in 'Urogynaecology and pelvic floor problems'. By the end of the training programme all trainees should theoretically have a basic understanding and be able to assess and manage straightforward pelvic floor problems. However, in practice it is unlikely that clinicians without further training would be competent to undertake pelvic floor surgery.

Advanced training skills modules (ATSMs)

In the last 2y of the training programme, trainees undertake ATSMs to develop additional skills in areas of interest. The 'Urogynaecology and vaginal surgery' ATSM is designed for trainees who want to practise urogynaecology as part of a generalist job. This module results in competence in primary prolapse surgery (vaginal repair, hysterectomy, sacrospinous fixation), urodynamics, and one primary continence procedure (usually mid-urethral sling).

There is now a 'Laparoscopic urogynaecology' module which can only be commenced in conjunction with or following completion of the 'Urogynaecology and vaginal surgery' module.

Subspecialty training

This is designed to give a comprehensive training programme in all aspects of pelvic floor dysfunction and includes urology, colorectal, and neurology modules in addition to urogynaecology. Laparoscopic urogynaecology is now a mandatory part of subspecialty training.

Resources

⅍ https://www.rcog.org.uk/en/careers-training/specialty-training-curriculum/

The multidisciplinary team (MDT)

▶ The role of the multidisciplinary team is well established in urogynaecology.

The draft NICE guidance 'Urinary incontinence and pelvic organ prolapse in women: management' (October 2018) proposes a model of clinical networks consisting of local and regional MDTs as outlined next.

Local MDT

Manages women with primary SUI, OAB, or prolapse.

The team should include:
- two urogynaecologists or urologists with expertise in female urology
- a urogynaecology, urology, or continence specialist nurse
- a pelvic floor specialist physiotherapist

and may also include
- a member of the care of the elderly team
- an occupational therapist
- a colorectal surgeon.

Regional MDT

Manages women with complex pelvic floor dysfunction, recurrent prolapse/continence issues, and mesh-related complications.

The team should include:
- a urologist with expertise in female urology
- a urogynaecology, urology, or continence specialist nurse
- a pelvic floor specialist physiotherapist
- a radiologist with expertise in pelvic floor imaging
- a colorectal surgeon with expertise in pelvic floor problems
- a pain specialist
- a healthcare professional trained in biofeedback

and may also include:
- a member of the care of the elderly team
- an occupational therapist
- a plastic surgeon.

The regional MDT may need access to the following services:
- psychology
- psychosexual counselling
- chronic pain management
- bowel symptom management
- neurology.

Rise and fall of mesh

- 1992—synthetic mesh used for sacrocolpopexy
- 1996—US FDA approves mesh for surgical management of SUI
- 2002—US FDA approves first mesh for surgical management of POP
- 2003—NICE approves TVT for SUI
- 2000s—multiple 'mesh kits' marketed, despite a lack of evidence for vaginal placement
- 2008—FDA issues a Public Health Notification alerting to rare complications associated with transvaginally placed mesh for SUI and POP
- 2012—FDA orders postmarketing surveillance. Several companies withdraw their products
- 2017—NICE withdraws approval for vaginal mesh for POP
- July 2018—UK suspension of all vaginal mesh (for POP and SUI) following the Cumberlege Report.

Mesh complications

- Reaction by the host foreign body
- Infection
- Chronic pain
- Mesh contracture
- Mesh exposure.

Mesh removal

- This is complex surgery requiring significant expertise.
- Surgical techniques include vaginal, abdominal, and laparoscopic approaches.
- Patients must be carefully counselled about the risk of the procedure including operative morbidity, failure of removal to resolve symptoms, and recurrence of the original pelvic floor disorder (prolapse or incontinence).

▶ It is difficult to ascertain the true incidence of mesh complications, and the risk of complication must be weighed against the potential benefit of using mesh implants. The risk appears highest with vaginally inserted mesh for POP.

▶ All complications must be reported to the MHRA.

The current position

At the time of writing all vaginally inserted meshes for SUI and POP remain 'paused' pending new guidance. Abdominally inserted meshes are excluded from this restriction but remain under high scrutiny.

The future of mesh surgery

NHS England has stated that the mesh 'pause' will remain in place until the following conditions are met:

- Surgeons should only undertake operations for SUI if they are appropriately trained, and only if they undertake operations regularly.
- Surgeons report every procedure to a national database.
- A register of operations is maintained to ensure every procedure is notified and the woman identified who has undergone the surgery.
- Reporting of complications via MHRA is linked to the register.
- Identification and accreditation of specialist centres for SUI mesh procedures, for removal procedures and other aspects of care for those adversely affected by surgical mesh.
- NICE guidelines on the use of mesh for SUI are published.

Resources

⅋ https://www.england.nhs.uk/mesh/

Index

Tables, figures, and boxes are indicated by an italic *t*, *f*, and *b* following the page number.

A

abdominal hysteropexy 75
mesh positioning 76*f*
technique 75*b*
ACE inhibitors, effect on
bladder function 56
adhesions 158
advanced training skills
modules (ATSMs) 168
Aldridge sling 46
allopurinol-induced
cystitis 94*b*
alpha-blockers, effect on
bladder function 56
ambulatory urodynamics
24
anal sphincter 142
management of faecal
incontinence 123*b*
obstetric injury
140*b*, 142–3
anatomy
pelvic floor 4, 5*f*
urinary tract 2
anorectal manometry 112*b*
anterior colporrhaphy 70*b*
anterior Delorme's
procedure 124
antibiotics
in catheter-associated
UTI 62
in recurrent UTI 92
anticholinergic
(antimuscarinic)
drugs 31*t*
in childhood
incontinence 148
contraindications 31*b*
effect on bladder
function 56
in overactive bladder
syndrome 30
side effects 30
apical prolapse 59
See also pelvic organ
prolapse
artificial anal
sphincters 123*b*
artificial urinary
sphincters 48
atrophic changes 152*b*

cystoscopic
appearance 15
augmentation
cystoplasty 32
autologous fascial sling 46
autonomic dysreflexia 132
average flow rate 18*f*

B

Baden–Walker
classification 60
bedwetting 148
biological grafts 172
bisacodyl 115
bladder 2
control of micturition 6
physiological changes of
pregnancy 138
symptoms in
pregnancy 138*b*
symptoms of POP 62
See also cystitis
bladder diverticulum 15
bladder injuries
at caesarean section 102
at laparoscopy 102–3
retroperitoneal 103
bladder pain syndrome
assessment 96
definition 96*b*
differential diagnosis 96
management 98*b*
prevalence and
aetiology 96
symptoms 96
bladder retraining (bladder
drill) 30
Boari flap 105
botulinum toxin A 31
bowel symptoms of
prolapse 62
brain lesions 130
bulk forming laxatives 115
Burch (open)
colposuspension 44

C

caesarean section
bladder injuries 102
ureteric injuries 103–4

calcium channel blockers,
effect on bladder
function 56
carcinoma *in situ* , cystoscopic appearance 15
cardinal ligament 4*b*, 5*f*
catheter-associated UTI
90
catheters 108
troubleshooting 109*t*
cerebral shock 130
childbirth 58
obstetric anal sphincter
injury 142–3
perineal trauma 140
postpartum urinary
retention 144–5
See also caesarean section
children
urinary incontinence 148
urinary tract infection
150
clean intermittent
self-catheterization 108
co-danthromer 115
coital incontinence 8
colorectal investigations
112*b*, 113*f*
colpocleisis 80
colposuspension 44
prolapse risk 58
compliance 6*b*, 21*b*
compressor urethrae 2
computed tomography
(CT) 12, 84*b*
constipation
assessment 115
causes 114
definition 114*b*
management 115
obstructed defaecation
syndrome 116
Parkinson's disease 130
continence
control of micturition 6
See also faecal incon-
tinence; urinary
incontinence
continence aids 36
contractility 21*b*
cyclophosphamide-induced
cystitis 94*b*

cystitis
  'interstitial' 96b
  non-bacterial 94b
  See also urinary tract
    infection
cystitis cystica 15
cystocele 59f
  surgery 70
  See also pelvic organ
    prolapse
cystography 84b, 85f
cystometry 20–2
  catheter positions 20f
  filling cystometry 20–2
  tests of provocation 22
  voiding cystometry 22
cystoscopy
  equipment 14
  indications 14
  relevant findings 15
  technique 14

D

darifenacin 31t
daytime frequency 8
defaecography (evacuating
  proctogram) 112b
dementia 130
demyelinating lesions 132
detrusor areflexia
  peripheral
    neuropathy 136
  sacral cord lesions 134
  spinal cord lesions 132
detrusor hyperreflexia
  brain lesions 130
  spinal cord lesions 132
detrusor myomectomy 32
detrusor overactivity
  (DO) 9b, 21
  urodynamic trace 29f
  See also overactive
    bladder (OAB)
    syndrome
diabetes, peripheral
  neuropathy 136
diuretics, effect on bladder
  function 56
D-mannose 92
drug-induced
  constipation 114
drug-induced cystitis 94b
drugs affecting bladder
  function 56
duloxetine 36
dysuria 8

E

ectopic ureter 52b
elderly people

laparoscopic surgery 158
urinary incontinence 154
endoanal ultrasonography
  112b, 113f
enterocele 59f
  surgery 72
  See also pelvic organ
    prolapse
episiotomy 140, 141f
evacuating
  proctogram 112b
examination 10
  in faecal incontinence 122
  in obstetric anal sphincter
    injury 142
  in obstructed defaecation
    syndrome 116
  in pelvic organ prolapse
    61f, 62
  in stress urinary
    incontinence 34
external urethral sphincter
  (compressor urethrae) 2

F

faecal incontinence
  assessment 122
  causes 122b
  management 123b
faecal softeners 115
fascial slings 46
fesoterodine 31t
filling cystometry 20–2
fistulae
  rectovaginal 126
  vesicovaginal 106–7
flow time 18f
Fowler's syndrome 55
frequency/volume charts 12
frontal lobe lesions 130
functional incontinence 52

G

giggle incontinence 148b
glycerine suppositories 115
gracilioplasty 123b

H

haematuria 88
Hasson entry 160
herpes zoster, sacral nerve
  involvement 136
hesitancy 8
history-taking 10
  in faecal incontinence 122
  in obstructed defaecation
    syndrome 116
  in overactive bladder
    syndrome 28

  in stress urinary
    incontinence 34
Hunner's ulcers 96b
hypnotics, effect on bladder
  function 56
hysterectomy
  prolapse risk 58
  ureteric injuries 103–4
  vaginal 74b
  vaginal vault prolapse 78

I

ileal conduits 110
iliococcygeus 4
imaging 12, 84b
  intravenous urography
    84b, 85f
  See also ultrasound imaging
incomplete (bladder)
  emptying, feeling of 9
incontinence, faecal
  assessment 122
  brain lesions 130
  causes 122b
  management 123b
incontinence, urinary 8
  brain lesions 130
  in children 148
  in the elderly 154
  terminology 8
  See also functional incon-
    tinence; mixed urinary
    incontinence; overflow
    incontinence; stress
    urinary incontinence
insensible (unconscious)
  urinary incontinence 8
intermittent stream 8
internal urethral sphincter 2
interstitial cystitis 96b
intravenous urography
  (IVU) 84b, 85f
intussusception 120
  surgery 124
investigations 12
  colorectal 112b, 113f
  cystoscopy 14
  in faecal incontinence 122
  urethral pressure
    profilometry 26
  urodynamic tests 16–24
  urological 84b
isotope renography 84b

K

ketamine-induced
  cystitis 94b
kidneys, physio-
  logical changes of
  pregnancy 138